Guide to Nursing's Social Policy Statement

Understanding the Profession from Social Contract to Social Covenant

by **Marsha D. M. Fowler**, PhD, MDiv, MS, RN, FAAN

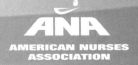

AMERICAN NURSES ASSOCIATION

American Nurses Association
Silver Spring, Maryland 2015

The American Nurses Association is the only full-service professional organization representing the interests of the nation's 3.1 million registered nurses through its constituent/state nurses associations and its organizational affiliates. The ANA advances the nursing profession by fostering high standards of nursing practice, promoting the rights of nurses in the workplace, projecting a positive and realistic view of nursing, and by lobbying the Congress and regulatory agencies on health care issues affecting nurses and the public.

American Nurses Association
8515 Georgia Avenue, Suite 400
Silver Spring, MD 20910-3492
1-800-274-4ANA
http://www.Nursingworld.org

Published by Nursesbooks.org
The Publishing Program of ANA
http://www.Nursesbooks.org

Cataloging-in-Publication Data on file with the Library of Congress

ISBN-13: 978-1-55810-615-4   SAN: 851-3481   10K   02/2016

First printing: July 2015. Second printing: February 2016.

Dedication

To nurses past
Who died in service, *victimes de leur dévouement*

To nurses present
Who live the nursing covenant

To nurses future
May pride of profession possess you

Contents

Acknowledgments

This work represents the disparate pieces from readings, experiences, friends, and career that I have brought together in building my own semi-unified field of knowledge. I am grateful to those who got me to this point in the journey, and to those who will continue to move me along the way. Particular thanks are due to Col. Martha Turner, PhD, RN-BC, USAF (Ret.) for support, suggestions, and efforts that were supererogatory (see chapter 4). I drew heavily from the work of Patricia Benner and am grateful for her contributions to the profession and for her friendship. Other friends along the way—Anne, Verena, Marilyn, Patricia, Marianne, Sheryl, Rick, Sonya—nurse–scholars all, who have been exemplars of the donative element of life and whose gifts have affected me deeply.

In the production of this work specifically, I am compelled to thank all of the librarians who have worked their information literacy wizardry on my behalf and without whose skill I could not have been nearly so productive. I am grateful as well for the editorial aid and abetment of Eric Wurzbacher at ANA, whose singular suggestions served to improve this work.

None of the above-named persons should be held complicit in any errors, gaps, loopholes, tautologies, logical fallacies, defects, or incomprehensibilities of this manuscript. If I have made a mess of it, know that I cooked all the sticky pudding myself.

It is my hope that this small contribution to the nursing literature will cause other nurses to think about nursing in new ways and to move beyond anything that I could even conceive, for the nursing profession and its covenant with humanity, but also for the goal of health for all.

Marsha D.M. Fowler, PhD, MDiv, MS, RN, FAAN
Pentecost 2015

Introduction
Where We Are Going and How We Intend To Get There

The American Nurses Association's *Nursing's Social Policy Statement* is a document about the relationship between the nursing profession and society, called a *social contract.* It is not about individual nurses and their practice, though its implications for practice are profound. Instead, this social policy statement is about how it is that there is a specific social need (health) that, in this case, leads to the creation and authorization of an occupational group called "nursing," to address that need, and what society and the state, or government, expect of this occupational group. However, this is not a one-sided relationship; therefore, this book is also about what nursing can expect from society and the state.

Here is a quick overview of this book's structure:

- Chapter 1: Social contracts, in theory and practice, including the nursing profession's social contract

- Chapter 2: Professions and what they are; nursing as a profession and how it got there

- Chapter 3: Understanding and fixing what's broken in professions; the idea of civic professionalism

- Chapter 4: Understanding and fixing what's broken in social contract; the implications of civic professionalism and cosmopolite professionalism; the idea of social covenant

- Afterword: Why the book's contents matter to nurses, with the feminization of HIV/AIDS as a case example

But nothing is ever quite so simple. The book begins with a consideration of social contract, the basic unit of the society–nursing relationship. The social contract is an unwritten social arrangement that authorizes and requires professions to meet specific needs, such as medical diagnosis, nursing care, legal defense, pastoral care, designing a building, and teaching our children to read, learn, and think. **Chapter 1** asks "What is a social contract?" The chapter will look at four successive formulations of social contract theory that, to some extent, build upon one another. It will also look at the important critiques of social contract theories. These theories have been critiqued for creating in-groups (those who benefit from the social contract) and out-groups (those who are excluded from or diminished within the social contract). The in-group has enduringly been white, privileged, land-owning males. The separate critiques identify out-groups as females, minority groups, and those with disabilities.

An additional critique is that social contract devalues caring and caring work, shoving it out of the public eye, into the private and hidden sphere. These critiques have implications for nursing both as a female-dominant profession and as a profession of caring work. In addition, nursing cares for many socially disadvantaged persons and groups who, according to the critiques, live outside the social contract. There is a discussion that looks at the differences between the social contract of medicine and that of nursing. The chapter concludes with a list of the social expectations that society has of nursing (such as competence and compassion, setting standards of practice), and that nursing has of society (such as protecting the RN title, licensure laws, social respect). These mutual expectations, sixteen in number, comprise the content of the social contract.

Chapter 1, and each of the subsequent chapters, includes a series of thought experiment questions. While the English phrase "thought experiment" has a long lineage in many areas of scholarship, I've used the German *Gedankenexperiment* (plural *Gedankenexperimente*) instead. Perhaps most famously used by Albert Einstein to describe his conceptual, approach to creating theory in physics, without the use of "lab experiments." A thought experiment can imaginatively open up potential avenues for further exploration. Accordingly, these *Gedankenexperimente* are not study questions on the chapter's contents. Rather, they are intended as imaginative, speculative, conjectural questions of the "What if…" and "Why couldn't we…" and "Suppose, instead, that…" variety of thinking, and thus are useful for personal reflection and group discussion in ways that might advance the content of the chapter.

IT'S A PERIOD THING…

Understanding two elements in this book may help you in your reading. First, a number of the quotations in the book (and in this chapter in particular) utilize British English spellings, and a few of the quotations are in "antique" English. The original spelling has been retained, and in the case of quotations using antiquated English, the capitalization of nouns has been retained. Second, some of the writings are from a period when nursing was an exclusively female profession, and thus refer to the nurse in feminine pronouns, and to all of humanity in masculine pronouns, or as "mankind" or "man". The quotes have not been altered to reflect current standards for inclusive language.

A social policy statement deals with the social contract that society and the state have with professions—in this book, with the nursing profession specifically. The second building block, then, is *professions*. **Chapter 2** asks "What is a profession?" It looks at a range of ways in which profession is defined. Modern nursing (after the Civil War) has always regarded itself as a profession, but society has not, so it has been something of a social struggle. The chapter begins with a look at the concepts of occupation, vocation, and calling before coming to different approaches to defining a profession. It then looks briefly at the role of professions in society.

Once we have looked at social contract, and at professions, it is time to begin putting them together in the third building block. **Chapter 3** begins with an examination of the new social context of the professions, specifically the shift from a manufacturing economy to a service and technological economy (called the *new economy*) and the new challenges that this presents for professions. It then looks at how professions are "broken" and how they might be "mended." This chapter relies heavily upon the works of William Sullivan and of Patricia Benner and colleagues, who call for a civic professionalism to reform professions and reclaim their social trust. Nursing has a distinctive position over other professions in claiming the highest level of social trust among all the professions.

Chapter 3 moves from a discussion of civic professionalism as applied to all professions to a closer look at nursing. Citizenship is discussed, as it has a long history in the nursing literature and is the basic seed that can be grown into civic professionalism. Sullivan and Benner and colleagues argue for specific approaches in professional and nursing education to prepare nurses as civic professionals; they specifically call for a multifaceted cognitive apprenticeship to accomplish this. *Cognitive apprenticeship* is an approach to teaching—learning that incorporates theory, clinical simulation, and clinical-expert mentored practice. The chapter looks at several barriers to preparing nurses as civic professionals, including the corporate ideals of the new economy and globalization, the loss of the liberal arts in higher education, the lack of knowledge about nursing's history, and the different education levels possessed by individuals entering the nursing practice. This chapter, too, concludes with a *Gedankenexperimente*.

The closing chapter, **Chapter 4**, adds its own building blocks and then brings the pieces together, which makes it the culmination of all the chapters as well as the most complex of the chapters. It begins with a focus on civic professionalism "beyond the bedside" as nurses work to transform health beyond our own society; that is, as nurses go global to make health for all a reality. It looks at the national focus of Sullivan and Benner and colleagues in their civic professionalism, and expands professionalism to include the global community in *cosmopolite professionalism*. Sullivan and Benner's cognitive apprenticeship is also extended to include education about what nurses do as well as what nurses are. So, there is a discussion of *doing* and *being* (introduced in Chapter 2) and how the expert, ethical nurse comes to wisdom, which is essential to both civic and cosmopolite professionalism. Cosmopolite professionalism requires nurses who set out to "change the world" for health to engage in social criticism and social change through social ethics. Chapter 4 also discusses social ethics and each of its three functions with illustrative examples, then proceeds to discuss cosmopolite professionalism, and social power structures and social meaning and value structures, and the need to balance the two structures. It examines the problems of the social contract as a framework and discusses three potential remedies in which nursing can participate: the capabilities approach, the political ethic of care, and the social covenant approach, with a consideration of the concept of the common good. The chapter concludes with *Gedankenexperimente.*

An extended example of the global feminization of HIV/AIDS is offered as the book's **Afterword** to bring specific, concrete meaning to the principles of the chapters. Here the discussion is limited to only one causal element, the structural adjustment policies of the World Bank and the International Monetary Fund. This is an example of how a poor nation's borrowing money can increase poverty and disease among its people. Borrowing also has negative effects upon education and employment. This afterword concludes with additional *Gedankenexperimente.*

The intent of this book is to discuss the building block concepts that are central to *Nursing's Social Policy Statement* in a way that, chapter by chapter, pulls them together. These are stacking blocks, so chapters should be read in sequence to the conclusion, where they will be brought together. This is not easy material, in large part because it deals with the nursing profession and society, not the individual nurse and society, and is therefore not material that often finds its way into basic nursing curriculum. It is not about clinical practice, but it has deep relevance for clinical practice. It is not about nursing research, but it has deep relevance for nursing research. It is not about nursing curriculum, but is has deep relevance for nursing curriculum.

THINKING ABOUT SIDEBARS...

Throughout the book there are sidebars, text boxes set off from the main text of the chapter. Unlike a "pull-quote" that you might see in a newspaper or magazine, in which a key sentence or quote is pulled from the text and highlighted graphically to entice you to read the article, sidebars serve a different function. These chapter sidebars are to provide you with additional material that explains a major concept (usually on a nearby page) or expands or otherwise develops the concept farther. They are here to offer you a moment to pause, reflect, to think—perhaps somewhat differently—about the main text material.

The road map of the book is as follows:

The social contract and broken social contracts ➜

The emergence of professions ➜

Repairing broken professions through civic professionalism ➜

Social contracts revisited ➜   Cosmopolite professionalism ➜

Healing the world

Nursing is called a helping profession and many of us went into nursing to help others. The social policy statement of our profession is about the multiple ways in which nursing helps others: through direct patient care, and by changing institutions, society, and global health. Nurses can be civic professionals and cosmopolite professionals and be active in any or all of these ways of helping. Nursing has a wide horizon, and the reader is invited to sail for any destination between here and nursing's farthest horizon, and to find good colleagues and companions along the way.

Marsha Fowler, PhD, MDiv, MS, RN, FAAN

Chapter 1.
Social Contract Theory
This Profession Called "Nursing,"
and its Rights, Privileges, and Obligations

Nursing's Social Policy Statement and Nursing's Social Contract

Nursing's Social Policy Statement (NSPS) is a document that articulates the parameters of the relationship between the profession of nursing and society.[1] It forms and frames both the basis for nursing's involvement with caring practices and the shape of society vis-à-vis health and health policy. It is not about the nurse–patient relationship, but instead about nursing as an entity within society, and how that relationship is to be understood, developed, and lived out by the profession as a whole.

While *Nursing's Social Policy Statement* is not about individual nurses, it is individual nurses who compose the profession, and thus all nurses are participants. It fundamentally roots the nursing–society relationship in social contract. Society recognizes a specific and specialized need—health—so it authorizes a group of workers to form an occupational group (called *nursing*) to address that need. Nursing, which has evolved from an occupational group into a profession, operates as a profession within the social contract.

Guide to Nursing's Social Policy Statement does not move section by section through the NSPS. Instead, this guide intends to explore the foundational concepts that underlie nursing's social contract, the central nervous system of the NSPS, so that its breadth, depth, and importance might be better understood. These concepts include social contract (Chapter 1); occupation, vocation, and profession (Chapter 2); citizenship, civic engagement, and civic professionalism (Chapter 3); and nursing's global health involvement through cosmopolite professionalism, nursing's social ethics, and social covenant (Chapter 4). *Nursing's Social Policy Statement* is inextricably tied to both *Nursing: Scope and Standards of Practice* (NSSP) and *Code of Ethics for Nurses with Interpretive Statements* ("the Code").[2,3,4] The NSSP and the Code are two of the sixteen elements of nursing's social contract. It is part of the task of this chapter to elucidate the ties that bind the three documents as foundational to nursing. To do so will require a brief consideration of the key findings of those philosophers who have most influenced our understanding of the social contract.

A Short History of Social Contract Theory: Understanding the Unwritten Social Arrangement It Creates

Any number of articles in medicine and nursing invoke the notion of social contract and presume an understanding of what that means. The writings then proceed with little or no substantive discussion of the origins, nature, or reciprocal obligations of a social contract. The concept of a social contract was developed in the fields of philosophy and political science, and as those discussions do not customarily make their way into nursing curricula, nursing students and nurses are left with little exposure to what a social contract is or how it functions. The general idea of a contract is that it is an enforceable agreement of mutual benefit made between two parties. Contracts may be written, as in suzerainty agreements of very ancient times between lords and vassals or vassal states, but more often today, social contracts are unwritten bilateral arrangements that contain conditions for both sides, and are subject to enforcement. Certain elements of social contracts may be written, such as the laws governing practice or the profession's code of ethics, but the social contract itself is an unwritten understanding. These contracts are always two sided and have expectations for each party of the contract, so in that sense, a social contract is no different from a written one. More specifically, a social contract is an abstract construct that comes out of philosophy, ethics, and political theory. That is to say that a social contract is a metaphor or heuristic device that is used for analysis, reflection, and argument; there is no formal legal contract involved.

Social contract has two formal components. The first explains how it is that *society* comes into being, and the second explains society then produces a state (or a *government*) and *a people* (as in "we the people" of the United States Constitution) that interact for mutual benefit. The first component has profound though more theoretical or less tangible implications for nursing. It is the second component that is more relevant for the discussion of nursing's relationship to and with society, as it delves into the discussion of what society needs from nursing and what nursing needs from society.

Theories of social contract reach back to antiquity though its strongest development occurs in the Enlightenment of the mid-1600s to mid-1700s. It threads its way through philosophy, religion, and politics. Early formulations are found in Plato's *Crito*[5],[6] and *Republic*, Book II,[7] and in Epicurus's *Principle Doctrines*.[8],[9] However, modern social contract theory owes its development to Thomas Hobbes, John Locke, Jean-Jacques Rousseau, and more recently, to John Rawls, who relies in part upon Immanuel Kant, and David Gauthier, who modifies Hobbes's theory. A very brief overview of the works of these theorists is given here, not to fully develop social contract theory, but to provide foundational information that can be used to situate nursing within the context of social contract theory. Social contract theory has also been subject to critique both by feminist theorists and critical race theorists. We will look at these critiques because they are important as critiques, but also because they intersect with nursing's concern for persons who are disadvantaged in society. We turn now to the theories of social contract and their successive formulations.

Hobbes: Overcoming a Life That is "solitary, poore, nasty, brutish, and short"

Thomas Hobbes (1588–1679), in his work *Leviathan* (1651), sets forth his political theory in two parts.[10] The first part argues that prior to the formation of society, individuals are in a *State of Nature*. In this state, persons are universally, necessarily, and exclusively self-interested, which causes them at all points to seek their own best interests. The State of Nature is a picture of rampant and exclusive self-interest wherein individuals are driven not only to satisfy their own desires and needs, but to avoid that which does not further the realization of their own desires. The State of Nature is a terrible place, as it is a state of brutality, fear, distrust, and danger, or, in Hobbes's own words, "continuall feare, and danger of violent death; And the life of man, solitary, poore, nasty, brutish, and short."[11] It is a state of unavoidable and perpetual warfare, as one seeks one's own best interests, even at the expense of another. But, Hobbes maintains that humans are also reasonable.

Because humans can be rational and reasonable, there is a way out by creating, with mutual agreement, a *commonwealth*—that is, *civil society*. It functions as a common-wealth because it serves the needs of all. However, for the commonwealth to function, and to keep rampant self-interest and warfare at bay, two things are necessary: enforceability of the "mutual covenants" or laws that govern a society, and a sovereign with the absolute authority to enforce the law. Hobbes argues that the only way people will fulfill their part of the covenant is through "the terror of some punishment greater than the benefit they expect by the breach of their covenant." [12] According to Hobbes, the establishment of the commonwealth is the only way to create this motivating fear: "Where there is no coercive power erected [created], that is, where there is no Commonwealth, there is no propriety [moral conformity], all men having right to all things. …The validity of covenants begins…with the constitution of a civil power sufficient to compel men to keep them." [13] The commonwealth

---

THINKING ABOUT THE COMMON-WEALTH…

Four states (Kentucky, Massachusetts, Pennsylvania, and Virginia) use the term commonwealth in their name, as in the Commonwealth of Virginia. The term has no actual legal meaning. Here it means both that the state was created by agreement of the people (not by the command of King George III), and that it serves the welfare and general good of all of its people. Sometimes commonwealth is written common-wealth, or even common wealth. It refers to the welfare, not the material wealth, of the people.

that is created is one in which "justice is the constant will of giving to every man his own."[14]

He argues that the sovereign (in his day, a monarch) has the absolute authority to enforce the laws generated under the social contract, and must be obeyed, even if he (rarely she) rules badly. The alternative is to return to the intolerable State of Nature, which no reasonable person would want. What one gives up by entering into the social contract is the right to do anything one desires and to seek one's own needs or desires at the expense of others. In addition, individuals become subject to punishment if they do so. Under the social contract, lives are protected, mutual benefit is secured, social cooperation is assured, agreements are kept, and laws are enforced. So, under the social contract, the brutal freedoms of the State of Nature are lost in exchange for socially secured goods such as a life that can be lived without fear, distrust, or warfare. It is not the State of Nature that is of greatest interest to nursing, but rather the second aspect of social contract, the concepts of government, civil society, rights, and mutuality, for it is from this portion of social contract theory that the rights and responsibilities of nursing arise.

Locke: Power to the People

Most social contract theorists employ some form of a State of Nature. However, John Locke (1632–1704) develops the notion of a social contract with a substantively different view of humankind than that held by Hobbes. The core of Locke's social contract theory is contained in his 1689 work *Two Treatises on Government* (the full title of which is *Two Treatises on Government: In the Former, The False Principles, and Foundation of Sir Robert Filmer, and His Followers, Are Detected and Overthrown. The Latter Is an Essay Concerning The True Original, Extent, and End of Civil Government*).[15] Hobbes holds that in the State of Nature there is neither justice nor injustice, that the State of Nature is amoral. For Hobbes, morality and law come into being with the creation of civil society. Locke is different in that he maintains that humankind is not engaged in a moral free-for-all in the State of Nature, that there are some limits even in the State of Nature. Morality exists in the State of Nature as humankind discerns and operates under a Law of Nature. In his understanding of the State of Nature, all persons are equal and are in a state of perfect freedom, free from interference by others. The Law of Nature creates a moral limit to that perfect freedom: Individuals may not exercise their freedom to pursue their own desires and needs at the expense of that same freedom for others. As Locke says, "how should I look to have any part of my desire herein satisfied, unless my self be careful to satisfie the like desire, which is undoubtedly in other Men, being of one and the same nature?"[16] So, this means that I may only satisfy my own desires insofar as I permit like desires to be satisfied by others. This pursuit of my own desires is governed by "rules and canons," moral rules, that I and all persons alike can know by reason.

As the Law of Nature guides human behavior in the State of Nature, in contrast to Hobbes, this state is not amoral. For Locke, property (including one's own body as property) and slavery are critical concepts: war ensues over issues of property or slavery, and once it begins, it is likely to continue. For Locke, "every Man has a Property in his own Person. This no Body has any Right to but himself."[17]

Our bodies are our own property and no one has a right to them. For Locke, this includes slavery as the appropriation of the body or property of another; for nursing, this might potentially ground self-determination in health care as derivative of "property rights" rather than respect for autonomy.

Locke also identifies property as that which is created by the labor of one's hands and combined with nature. The creation of private property—that is, real property (land)—and its acquisition removes it from that which is held in common. In the archaic language of Locke,

> The Labour of his Body, and the Work of his Hands, we may say, are properly his. What-soever then he removes out of the State that Nature hath provided, and left it in, he hath mixed his Labour with, and joyned to it something that is his own, and thereby makes it his Property.[18]

In the State of Nature, there is no authority that enforces one's property rights. The creation of civil society and government is therefore required in order to create laws that protect the life, health, liberty, and possessions of all, thereby in theory preventing war over theft of land or possessions, or enslavement.[19]

Locke also differs dramatically from Hobbes in how he views the relationship between society and government. For Hobbes, the sovereign is absolute ruler who must be obeyed even when he rules badly. Locke, however, sees the people as having a right, perhaps even an obligation, to overthrow the ruler or government when it becomes tyrannical or fails to serve the commonwealth. The people then have a right to put a new government in place. If Locke's view sounds familiar—it is. It deeply influenced Thomas Jefferson and the leaders of the American Colonies in their decision to break away from the tyrannical King George III and to create a constitution that protects life, liberty, the pursuit of happiness, and property. It should also be noted that Locke viewed the land as the possession of those who worked it, that is, those who combined labor (plowing and planting) with the raw resources of nature (the soil). In his schema, one that is culturally bound to a European, agrarian understanding of society, Native Americans never owned the land as their property because they did not till and plant it.[20] It belonged, instead, to those who farmed it. This too informed the early founders of the United States and was used as a justification for taking Native American lands without recompense or permission. One can see that social disparities, which would eventually create health disparities, are present even at the very beginnings of the creation of the United States from the British Colonies.

Rousseau: Social Contract Gone Wrong and the More Perfect Union

Jean-Jacques Rousseau (1712–1778) discusses social contract in two different ways. The first discussion lays out his description of the social contract gone wrong. This is found in his *Second Discourse*, also known as the *Discourse on the Origin and Foundation of Inequality Among Mankind* (1753).[21] It was a radical and shocking critique of the ills of Western society in his day, particularly the economic disparities that created classes of the poor and the rich. He then follows this critique with a corrective, a normative or prescriptive version of the social contract, found in his treatise *The Social Contract* (1762).

Rousseau, too, employs the device of a State of Nature in which people are free, equal, and rational. However, Rousseau envisions them as independent, solitary persons, with simple needs, capable of meeting their own needs without relational ties. For Rousseau, it is a picture of humankind evolving into ever larger groups. As humankind evolves in this state of nature, the family develops into a "little society,"[22] in which women are subordinated to patriarchy, solitariness disappears, language develops, enabling cooperation and the creation of communities, and cooperation begins, giving rise to leisure. These are all seen as good things by Rousseau.

As population increases, divisions of labor develop and people become less able to satisfy all of their own needs, becoming instead reliant upon others for the provision of specific needs. So the housewife needs the miller for flour, the farmer comes to the blacksmith for a plow, the blacksmith needs the miner

---

THINKING ABOUT THE STATE OF NATURE...

Is humankind intrinsically good, or intrinsically evil? This question sits underneath discussions of the State of Nature in the different social contract theories. Think back to William Golding's famous novel *Lord of the Flies*, for which he was awarded the Nobel Prize in Literature. The novel contains many of the themes of State of Nature discussions in social contract theories, themes such as human nature, individual self-interest, and the common good. In *Lord of the Flies*, a group of preadolescent, well-educated, civilized British boys are marooned on an uninhabited, paradise-like island. The story starts out well enough as they set about establishing a form of order and governance that will help them survive and be rescued. The situation devolves disastrously into savagery before they are actually rescued. The novel is a good read, though a hard read, and useful for reflecting on social contract.

for ore, the miner needs both the beck (pick-axe maker) and the sawyer (lumber-maker); they all might need a bullard to write a letter…and so on. People grow less and less self-reliant and more interdependent upon the labor of others. The development of a concept of private property (my land, my plow, my pickaxe, etc.) follows, and with it the development of greed, competition, vanity, deceit, and a host of vices, in addition to inequality, social classes, and ultimately warfare; "…in short," Rousseau writes, "competition and rivalry on the one hand, opposition of interests on the other, and always the hidden desire to profit at the expense of someone else. All these ills are the first effect of property and the inseparable offshoot of incipient inequality."[23] It is private property that is pivotal in making civil society and government necessary. Those who have property want government to protect their property, to advantage them, and to cement inequality. In Rousseau's opinion, it is also private property for which "the vices that make social institutions necessary are the same ones that make their abuses inevitable."[24] This is the dysfunctional, dystopian social contract that he describes in the *Second Discourse*.

As a corrective, Rousseau envisions a different kind of social contract (sometimes called a *social compact*). In his normative reenvisioning of the social contract, communities come together to form a society and everyone places "his person and all his power in common under the supreme direction of the general will; and as one, we receive each member as an indivisible part of the whole."[25] One people, a people is formed to become one society, uniting individual wills to create one general will, enabling all to live together. It is the general will that decides and directs the actions of the society. For Rousseau, this act "whereby a people is a people…is the true foundation of society."[26] In becoming a (one) people, individuals give up the liberties of the State of Nature, instead, transferring their freedoms to the people as a collective body. This collective body becomes sovereign, creating a collective or general will that seeks to work for the good and benefit of all those who compose the people. So, as one people, the individual will becomes a general will that both defines and seeks the common good. The people are sovereign and through a democratic process form a government that executes the general will of the people. That general will is always to be determined through a democratic process. Ideally, in Rousseau's democracy, each and every citizen participates in deciding the laws that will govern the people.

And yet, not everyone participates in shaping the general will. Low voter turnout in elections indicates a failure of the one people to participate in shaping the general will. In addition, it should be noted that in the 1700s, democracy in the American Colonies and early United States was somewhat less than "democratic." While considered citizens, white women could not vote until 1920, some 144 years later. African American women still faced difficulties voting through the 1960s (particularly in the South, where state laws essentially prohibited most from voting).[27] In fact, women, those under the age of majority, white men who did not own land (real property), indentured servants, slaves, and Native Americans could not vote in colonial America. Only freemen could vote. Historically, a freeman was: (a) not a slave, (b) a member of a municipal corporation (a city or a borough) who possessed full civic rights, especially the right to vote, and (c) a freeholder (landowner).[28] Until relatively recently, these were the only people allowed to decide what constituted the general will and thus the common good.

This Lockean sense of a social contract and Rousseau's notion of the people deeply informs the U.S. Constitution. The Preamble to the *Constitution of the United States* (1789) states:

> We the People of the United States, in Order to form a more perfect Union, establish Justice, insure domestic Tranquility, provide for the common defence, promote the general Welfare, and secure the Blessings of Liberty to ourselves and our Posterity, do ordain and establish this Constitution for the United States of America. [29]

In only 52 words, the concepts of the one people, the common good ("general welfare"), the absence of the strife of the State of Nature (domestic tranquility), liberty and justice as part of the common good, and more, are present in the Preamble. These concepts are then expanded in the Constitution itself. While social contract is a philosophical and political concept, it finds real life expression in the way in which the United States was envisioned and conducts its life today. More importantly, as will be seen shortly in the critiques of social contract, who does or does not participate in constituting the general will, and thus determining the common good, has profound implications for the structure of the healthcare system, healthcare delivery, and health disparities.

Rawls: The Two Principle Prenuptial Agreement to the Social Contract

Social contract theory had lain fallow until John Rawls broke new soil with the publication of *A Theory of Justice* in 1972.[30] Rawls employs Immanuel Kant's understanding of humankind as rational beings, able to reason from a universal point of view—that is, a point of view from which all (all = universal) rational persons can argue impartially Rawls develops his own version of the State of Nature, a theoretical construct he terms the *Original Position*, that is characterized by a Veil of Ignorance. Under the Veil of Ignorance, I do not know who I am; I have no knowledge of my sex, age, race, socioeconomic status, education, or even what I might need or desire. Without this knowledge I am rational and disinterested (not influenced by my own self-interests) and can discover what justice requires and what is fair. Rawls maintains that everyone and anyone behind the Veil of Ignorance would choose the same rational, disinterested, universal principles of justice, in agreement with all others arguing from the same original position. We would all choose fairly. In a sense, it is like dividing a pie. If you are slicing the pie and you don't know which piece will be yours, you will cut the pie in even pieces. Rawls maintains that his theory is one of justice defined as fairness.[31] From this original position, persons can reason to what is just and fair. Justice then helps us decide what is needed in order to live together as a society.

Rawls describes the two principles of justice that would arise universally from the original position behind the Veil of Ignorance:

> The first requires equality in the assignment of basic rights and
> duties, while the second holds that social and economic inequalities,
> for example inequalities of wealth and authority, are just only if they
> result in compensating benefits for everyone, and in particular for
> the least advantaged members of society.[32]

The first principle accords individuals maximum liberty compatible with like liberty for all.[33] We saw this similarly in Locke: maximum freedom compatible with like freedom for all. The second principle permits social and economic inequalities *only* if such inequalities also serve to better the situation of the least well off in society.[34] This is Rawls's *difference principle*.[35] Choosing in this way would mean that if, when the Veil of Ignorance lifts, I find myself among the least advantaged in society, even despite difference (inequality), my lot is still improved. His argument is not specifically about wealth, and not about a redistribution of wealth, though it is, in part, about sharing in wealth. For Rawls, there are primary social goods to which all are entitled, such as liberty, opportunity, justice, and so forth. The maximization of these goods is just and should be promoted. Rawls is concerned, in part, that the circumstances into which one is born are random and that some win and some lose in the birth lottery. Circumstances will dictate, for example, whether one is born to a wealthy, aristocratic family, or to a sharecropper family—think, feudal lord

---

THINKING ABOUT SOCIAL STARTING POINTS…

There is an old saying about being "born with a silver spoon in his mouth." References to silver spoons appear in the songs of the Gershwins though Creedence Clearwater Revival and the Beatles to Lily Allen. What these silver spoons have in common is a reference to persons who are born into inherited wealth, privilege, and a life of ease. Their starting point in life lacks the struggle that others acquire by virtue of their own perhaps plastic spoon starting point that these musicians sing about. John Rawls' theory is concerned about the lack of fairness of social starting points, the social position to which one is born. Rawls tries to soften the blow to persons born to disadvantaged positions by insisting that the least well off in society ought not suffer in circumstances where the rich get richer. He does not oppose the rich getting richer but insists that if the rich get richer, justice as fairness demands that the poor must become better off too.

versus serf. In addition, some will be born who can run faster and jump higher, sing better, write better, or think more abstractly—think Kobe Bryant or Albert Einstein. The natural lottery determines not only the circumstances into which one is born but also the abilities that one is born with—randomly and arbitrarily. For Rawls, these natural assets and endowments are to be used in such a way that they benefit all. So those with better social circumstances or with stronger natural abilities may use their natural assets to improve their own lot, so long as in doing so it contributes to the good of the less well off in society. As Rawls states, "those who have been favored by nature, whoever they are, may gain from their good fortune only on terms that improve the situation of those who have lost out."[36]

Rawls's highly abstract theory of justice addresses the conditions that must exist prior to establishing a social contract, for only these conditions will in the end make for a social contract that is just and fair. These conditions would prevent the creation of Rousseau's first description of the social contract gone wrong by placing limits on political and social organization that are necessary to create a just society. Rawls's concept of justice as fairness, as well as Kant's perspective on autonomy as rational self-legislation, receive considerable attention in the bioethics literature as well as the nursing ethics literature, specifically in considerations of respect for patient autonomy (patient self-determination), access to health care, and the structure of healthcare systems.

Feminists, Critical Race Theorists, and Social Outliers: In-Groups and Out-Groups

The focus of this chapter is on the rights, privileges and obligations of nursing that are generated by its social contract rather than on critiquing social contract. Even so, it would be unwise to bypass some of the substantive critique that has been lodged against it, particularly because it has implications for those who are socially disadvantaged, and ultimately affects ways in which one may think about health disparities.

Social contract theory has not escaped critique by feminist and critical race theorists or those who work in the domain of intersectionality. Critical theories, as a category, engage in social criticism to the end of social change. They go beyond being descriptive or explanatory to actually seeking change. Critical race theory, a subtype of critical theory, specifically examines society at the intersections of race, law, culture, and power. Intersectionality is often used by critical theorists to examine the interconnections of socially constructed categories (such as race, ethnicity, class, gender) and socially constructed prejudices (such as racism, sexism, ageism, homophobia, handicapism, xenophobia, classism, and the like) and how they create social-structural systems of oppression, domination, discrimination, and disadvantage. That is, they look at how social constructs intersect and are used to create or perpetuate structural injustices.[37, 38]

Feminist theorists have provided a range of potent critiques of the contract theories of Hobbes, Locke, Rousseau, and Rawls, and of Kant and others as well. Carole Pateman,[39] Eva Kittay,[40] Annette Baier,[41] Jean Hampton,[42] Jean Elshtain,[43] Virginia Held,[44] Joan Tronto, and Susan Okin[45] are prominent among the many feminist theorists who have critiqued social contract theory.[46] Their critiques have been of sufficient substance that they are now taken into account by contemporary "contractarians" (whose roots are in Hobbes) and "contractualists" (whose roots are in Rousseau), both of whom advocate contract theory. While there are several somewhat differing critiques, they do intersect, working together to provide a holistic critique.

Pateman is a leading critic of social contract theory. Her critique is extensive, nuanced, and complex. For our purposes here the thrust of her argument is that "the classic theorists had left a legacy of problems about women's incorporation into, and obligation within, civil society that contemporary arguments failed to acknowledge." She argues that "the social contract presupposed the sexual contract, and that civil freedom presupposed patriarchal right."[47] Her essential point is that "contract is seen as the paradigm of free agreement. But women are not born free; women have no natural freedom. ...Sexual difference is political difference; sexual difference is the difference between freedom and subordination."[48]

The first part of her argument is that the original contract was made by men and constructed in such a way as to privilege men and to grant men freedom. It was at the same time a contract that brought women under the domination of men as a contractual norm that reflected the social norms of the day. She proceeds to discuss a variety of ways in which women are made unequal and denied voice by the social contract:

> The original pact is a sexual as well as a social contract: it is sexual in the sense of patriarchal—that is, the contract establishes men's political right over women—and also sexual in the sense of establishing an orderly access by men to women's bodies [through the

---

THINKING ABOUT CRITICAL THEORY...

Critical theories, as a family of theories, engage in a reflective assessment and critique of society and culture. The tools of critical theories are composed of a wide range of both social sciences and humanities. A theory is a critical theory to the extent that it seeks "emancipation from slavery," acts as a "liberating...influence," and "is not just a research hypothesis which shows its value in the ongoing business of men; it is an essential element in the historical effort to create a world which satisfies the needs and powers of human beings."[71] Critical theory is not simply analysis and critique. It is also possessed of a reformist bias, often with a social justice concern at its heart. Critical theory, whether feminist-, race- or abilities-focused (see also pg. 94), has an agenda: the critique of society and culture in order to change the world to move it toward meeting the needs of *all* humankind.

marriage contract]. …Contract is far from being opposed to patriarchy; contract is the means through which patriarchy is constituted.[49]

Thus women are denied freedom from the start of the social contract. But she goes further:

> Patriarchal civil society is divided into two spheres, but attention is directed to one sphere only. The story of the social contract is treated as an account of the creation of the public sphere of civil freedom. The other, private, sphere is not seen as politically relevant. Marriage and the marriage contract are, therefore, also deemed politically irrelevant.[50]

She and other feminists note that social contract consigns women and women's work—caring—to the private sphere, the sphere of "dependency care"[51] or "intimate labor" that is hidden from view and poorly compensated or not compensated at all.[52] Tronto observes that women in the 18th century sought new public roles that "had to be contained and were contained by arguing that women naturally belonged within the household. Another side of this picture is also important: the locating of moral sentiments within the household."[53] She asserts that women's desire to act in the social sphere, coupled with their capacity to reason, could not be contained and so threatened the status quo. By framing a social construct of differing spheres and types of activity for men and women, women were able to be contained: "Women were creatures of sentiment, best exercising their virtue in the context of the household. …As women became increasingly identified with feeling, men were increasingly left free to be identified with reason. It was a small leap, then, for Kant to exclude women and to ensconce men within the possibility of fully and true moral life."[54] From here it easy to imagine where this went in terms of the place of nurses and nursing in society.

Women are subordinated in the original male-constructed social contract, relegated to the hidden sphere in society, and their labors are devalued. In addition, as the purveyors of care and caring work, women fall outside of the rationalistic Kantian configurations of the moral life. For Kant, autonomy consists in rational self-legislation. Women, socially identified with sentiment, not reason, did not fulfill the Eurocentric "perspective of masculinity" that philosophers of the 18th and 19th centuries were promulgating. Christine DiStephano, in her 1991 book *Configurations of Masculinity*, demonstrates that a number of important modern moral philosophers developed their theories with a normative understanding of "mankind" that contained a normative understanding of masculinity.

Taking a somewhat different approach, Tronto, Held, Baier and other feminist theorists working in "care ethics" maintain that the disinterested, dispassionate, disembodied, universal person of Rawls, Kant, and others does not provide an adequate account of our moral, social or political obligations and that the State of Nature of contract theories does not give an adequate account of humanity. For example, for Hobbes, persons in the state of nature are radically individual without affiliative–affectional ties, and driven by fear. Even as a logical and fictional construct, it is an inadequate view that leaves out affectional bonds, caring for one another, dependency, and more. Held maintains that "various philosophers claim that even morality itself is best understood in contractual terms" but that

> As expressions of normative concern…contractual theories hold out an impoverished view of human aspiration. To see contractual relations between self-interested or mutually disinterested individuals as constitution the paradigm of human relations is to take a certain historically specific conception…as representative of humanity. And it is, many feminists are beginning to agree, to overlook or to discount in very fundamental ways the experience of women.[55]

While social contract does not specify a system of ethics or duties, it nonetheless contains normative elements that impinge upon prevailing theories of ethics and their relationship to nursing, as well as the way that nursing conceives its moral concepts, values, ideals and obligations. For example, nursing ethics necessitates a view of the person—one that is not adequately explained by the social contract theories. That is, a central moral claim of nursing is that the patient is a person of worth and dignity, deserving of care and compassion,

---

THINKING ABOUT DISADVANTAGED GROUPS…

Social concern for the ways in which society's social structures advantage some and disadvantage others is a matter of dawning awareness. In the 1800s, issues of the position of African-Americans and women surfaced—and persist. Society did not, then, have an awareness of the ways in which older adults, persons with disabilities, some immigrants were disadvantaged by the status quo. That awareness would not dawn until some decades later. The critique of social contract theory is that it either omits some minority groups from the contract or it fixes some groups in a subordinate position within the social contract. Pateman, Kittay, Baier, Hampton, Elshtain, Held, Tronto, Okin and others (see that discussion starting on page 11) have all critiqued social contract theory for its subordination of women within the contract. Mills extends the feminist critique to include the ways in which the social contract disadvantages racial minorities. Silvers and Francis extend the critique even farther to explore ways in which social contract disadvantages persons with disabilities, "outliers in society." Women, racial and ethnic minorities, persons with disabilities—these are social minorities. They are not necessarily numeric minorities; however social minorities they are differentiated, defined, and in both covert and overt ways, disadvantaged by the social contract. Perhaps one day the light of awareness will next dawn for the nation's largest minority: minors.

without regard for personal attributes or socioeconomic status. The social contract theories look to avoid strife, protect property, etc., and contain a descriptive and restricted view of human desires or interactions, but not a full descriptive view of persons per se. That is, they only describe one aspect of the person (e.g., self-interest, fear, envy, etc.) and do not give a full account of humanity individually or collectively. Tronto's work is of particular note in that it attempts to make a political argument for an ethic of care, in effect to modify if not radically change the boundaries between politics, morality, and caring practices, in effect to change the social contract.[56]

Charles Mills, inspired by Carole Pateman's *Sexual Contract*, extends a similar critique based on race, that he terms the *Racial Contract*:

> But the peculiar contract to which I am referring, though based on the social contract tradition that has been central to Western political theory, is not a contract between everybody ("we the people"), but between just the people who count, the people who really are people ("we the white people"). So it is a Racial Contract.[57]

As feminist theorists note the exclusion of women from the social contract (though some beginning changes in that contract have been acknowledged), so too, Mills notes the exclusion of a number of people groups and issues from the social contract:

> The "Racial Contract," then, is intended as a conceptual bridge between two areas now largely segregated from each other: on the one hand, the world of mainstream (i.e., white) ethics and political philosophy, preoccupied with discussions of justice and rights in the abstract, on the other hand, the world of Native American, African American, and Third and Fourth World political thought, historically focused on issues of conquest, imperialism, colonialism, white settlement, land rights, race and racism, slavery, jim crow, reparations, apartheid, cultural authenticity, national identity, indigenismo, Afrocentrism, etc. These issues hardly appear in mainstream political philosophy, but they have been central to the political struggles of the majority of the world's population. Their absence from what is considered serious philosophy is a reflection not of their lack of seriousness but of the color of the vast majority of Western academic philosophers.[58]

Using Pateman and Mills as a foundation, Silvers and Francis posit that persons with disabilities also become outliers in social contract theory:

Commentators concerned about justice for women and racial minorities have argued that social contract theory is inherently flawed. Far from offering a firm foundation on which to build comprehensive concurrence about justice, these critics contend, the contract model enables mutual agreement only within the boundaries of an "in-group/out-group" frame. Pateman, for example, has argued that the contract model reaches only a restrictive mutuality that privileges men and denies recognition to women. Mills has similarly claimed that contract theory positions African Americans at a disadvantage where justice is concerned. These authors contend that the social contract model places "outliers," either individually or collectively, in "out-groups" beyond the reach of equal justice. More recent versions of the "outlier problem" charge that social contract theory stands between people with disabilities and justice.[59]

Kittay, Jennings, and Wasunna emphasize the failure of social contract theory to take account of dependency. Their particular concern is for long-term care, especially long-term care of frail elderly persons; they question the adequacy of social contract to support dependency care in general and the needs of the frail elderly specifically:

> As a result of feminist scholarship, we have come to understand that the invisibility of human dependency and dependency care is in part a product of a private–public distinction that places a premium on the public and relegates issues of dependency to the private domain. But we can ask if the private/public distinction is itself a product of our deep denial of the inevitability of human dependency. Within the theoretical literature and political life of the Western industrialized nations, at least, we are captives of the myth of the independent, unembodied subject—not born, not developing, not ill, not disabled and never growing old—that dominates our thinking about matters of justice and questions of policy.[60]

THINKING ABOUT INTERSECTIONALITY...

The world's most perfect, amazing, and useful mobile phone with the world's most perfect, amazing, and useful apps is of little use to real people if the engineers do not take into account the fact that humans drop things, that winters are cold, summers are hot, and children throw things down the toilet. The most perfect electronics have to be able to withstand the use and abuse of real humans in a real environment. Their development for humans cannot ignore human reality. Intersectionality and intersectional theories try to take account of real humans and human reality by looking at factors that intersect and influence one another—like race, class and gender. Any study of social contract and nursing must consider real nurses and the real world of nursing—particularly its intersections with gender, culture, and power.

Thus, the discourse continues from successive formulations and reformulations of social contract theory to its critique by feminists, critical race theorists, and intersectionalists concerned about persons with disabilities or the frail elderly—and nurses. What begins as an abstraction, a fiction with no direct application, in the end has implications for the real-life professional concerns of nurses.

Social Contract and Health Care: Medicine Is Not Nursing

A social contract applies to the whole of society and its members. However, there seem to be levels of social contract. As examples of the appropriation of social contract to a global health setting, Kittay, Jennings and Wasunna, as noted above, address long-term care of the frail elderly as a global contractual issue, and Ooms and colleagues, write about "a global social contract to reduce maternal mortality."[61] In general social contract is applied to one nation and its people. And yet, as we note in Pateman and Mills, there is a range of large, unwritten social contracts for segments of society, including the marriage contract, the sexual contract, the racial contract—and somewhat more circumscribed social contracts contract between society and professions. In the realm of economics and finance, Donaldson and Dunfee make a distinction between macro- and microcontracts, but the microcontracts refer to smaller economic communities, not to professions.[62] There is no clear discussion of the movement from a social contract with the whole of society to these smaller contracts with specific groups within society in the healthcare literature. Despite the lack of theoretical justification in the literature for that development, both medicine and nursing have long laid claim to a social contract with society.

Medicine in the United States began to form as a modern profession earlier than nursing. Until such time as a guild is formed, an occupational group cannot speak of a social contract. For medicine, this occurred in the mid-1800s; modern nursing in the United States began to coalesce as an occupational group in the later 1800s and more especially after the formation of the American Nurses Association (ANA) in 1900 and the establishment of its offices in the 1920s. There is, in the first code of ethics of the American Medical Association (AMA), founded in 1847, an implicit understanding that a social contract exists

---

THINKING CONTRACTUALLY...

Both medicine and nursing talk about having a social contract; meaning a contract with society. *Social contract* is a also metaphor for a general social arrangement. Social contract does not have provisions; it is not specific in the sense of, say, sales or rentals or service contracts. However, like any everyday contract, there are two parties involved (nursing and society) and both parties have to do something to meet their contractual obligations. Here, society contracts with "nursing" to provide health care, and nursing contracts with society to set its own standards of practice and education.

between medicine and society. Chapter III, article 1, section 1 of the AMA *Code of Medical Ethics* (1847) states:

> As good citizens, it is the duty of physicians to be ever vigilant for the welfare of the community, and to bear their part in sustaining its institutions and burdens: they should also be ever ready to give counsel to the public in relation to matters especially appertaining to their profession, as on subjects of medical police, public hygiene, and legal medicine. It is their province to enlighten the public in regard to quarantine regulations,-the location, arrangement, and dietaries of hospitals, asylums, schools, prisons, and similar institutions, - in relation to the medical police of towns, as drainage, ventilation, &c., - and in regard to measures for the prevention of epidemic and contagious diseases; and when pestilence prevails, it is their duty to face the danger, and to continue their labours for the alleviation of the suffering, even at the jeopardy of their own lives.[63]

This section of the 1847 *Code of Medical Ethics* indicates the physician's wider responsibilities beyond those owed to an individual patient. Other elements commonly associated with a social contract are found elsewhere in that AMA *Code of Medical Ethics*. However, medicine, elsewhere, has explicitly adopted social contract as the model of physician–society relationship. Wynia asserts that social contract had a particular appeal to American medicine:

> It was the American medical profession that, in the mid-19th century, created the first national set of ethical and practice standards. Eventually, similar standards were almost universally accepted, thereby creating the modern concept of the medical profession. American physicians were primed for the task of creating a fullfledged profession for several reasons. Perhaps most important was the Americans' attraction to the notion of a social contract—a notion conceived by French, English, and Scottish Enlightenment thinkers, but implemented most fully in the young American republic, created by rebels against inegalitarian classism. In the United States, people were to relate as equals. Social relations were to be built upon moreor-less explicit contracts between willing parties, not such nebulous notions as noblesse oblige or gentlemanly honor. This way of thinking led to the desire to specify the terms of social relations. In medicine, this specification would take the form of a written code of ethics.[64]

Cruess and Cruess, who have written extensively on social contract in medicine, have identified three sets of expectations based on "three interlocking societal components…patients and patient groups as well as the 'public'…health-care managers, the state, government…departments…and the…medical profession and 'professional bodies.'"[65] They develop a list of societal expectations of medicine as well as medicine's expectations of society, deriving the list from their definition of a profession. Government's expectations of medicine are:

- Assured competence of physicians
- Morality, integrity, honesty
- Compliance with healthcare system—laws and regulations
- Accountability: performance, productivity, cost-effectiveness
- Transparency in decision-making and administration
- Participation in team health care
- Source of objective advice
- Promotion of the public good

Medicine's expectations of government are:

- Trust sufficient to meet patient's needs
- Autonomy sufficient to exercise judgment and self-regulation
- Healthcare system: value-laden, equitable, adequately funded and staffed, reasonable freedom within system
- Role in developing health policy
- Monopoly through licensing laws
- Rewards: nonfinancial (respect, status), financial[66]

THINKING ABOUT PROFESSIONAL SELF-REGULATION…

One attribute of professions is that they are self-policing to ensure that those who avail themselves of the professional's service will are getting competent service and will not be harmed. Self-policing, however, has been failing abysmally. The bioethical emphases on respect for patient self-determination, informed consent, and patient voluntariness arose as a response to the Nazi medical atrocities of World War II. These were brought to light in 1947, at the trial of 27 Nazi physicians (Annas and Grodin, 1992). Horrific, radically evil, and often lethal experiments were conducted on non-consenting human prisoners. Nurses participated in the conduct of unconscionable medical experimentation on unwilling prisoners, and were complicit in the medical killings in Nazi Germany (Froth, 2013a; 2013b). In 1966, Henry Beecher published his landmark paper on ethics in human research in the United States (Beecher, 1966). He identifies twenty-two medical research projects that were conducted from prestigious universities and published in respected medical journals, that were deeply, even frighteningly, ethically questionable. Nurses were directly and indirectly involved in a number of these experiments as well. Self-policing remains an ideal.

As would be true of nursing as well, the terms of these expectations are articulated in the profession's code of ethics and practice/education standards. Social contract, a profession's ethics, and its standards of education and practice are interrelated but far from coextensive.

Nursing too employs the device of a social contract to explicate its relationship with society, including the expectations of nursing by society and those that nursing has for society. A set of reciprocal expectations for nursing and society can be drawn from *Nursing's Social Policy Statement*, the *Code of Ethics for Nurses with Interpretive Statements*, the definition of nursing, the metaparadigm concepts of nursing, and the nursing literature on nursing as a profession, ethics, and caring. Medicine and nursing differ in a wide range of professional, philosophical, ethical, social, and political respects, yet, because they both interact with health and illness (and each other), there is both overlap and difference between the lists. The difficulty of extrapolating expectations from a definition of *profession,* as Cruess and Cruess have done, is that such definitions have been critiqued as being descriptive, rather than normative, in which case the list that is generated is tautological. We shall look at the concept of profession in the next chapter, but for now we turn to the reciprocating expectations between society and nursing.

The 16 Elements of the Social Contract: Reciprocal Expectations Between Nursing and Society

Nursing's social contract can be expressed in terms of 16 elements of reciprocal expectations: nine compose professional societal expectations of nursing, seven nursing's of society. Together, these elements constitute the social contract between nursing and society.

Society's Expectations of Nursing within the Social Contract

Within the social contract, society has expectations or for the obligations that nursing must meet as a profession. Much of society's faith in nursing rests upon its perceived and real faithfulness in meeting these obligations. Insofar as nursing meets these expectations, social trust is built. Were nursing to fail to meet these expectations, society would have several avenues of action to pursue, such as rescinding some of nursing's privileges, increasing the regulation and oversight of the profession, or taking control of portions of professional activity previously under the autonomous control of the profession. Nursing, however, gives evidence both of meeting these expectations and of a high level of social trust: "For the past 13 years, the public has voted nurses as the most honest and ethical profession in America in the Gallup poll. This year [12/2014], 80 percent of Americans rated nurses' honesty and ethical standards as 'very high' or 'high,' 15 percentage points above any other profession."[67]

That trust has been hard won. While it relies upon the belief that nurses are honest and uphold ethical standards, that reliance is meaningless unless the public also believes that nurses know what they are doing and that they exercise competence and skill. Honesty, ethical standards, and competence are a part of the societal expectations of nursing. More specifically, those expectations include the following general expectations.

1. Caring Service: That nursing care will be given with compassion and will preserve the dignity and recognize the worth of patients without prejudice. From this flows an expectation of patient participation in care decisions and self-determination. Caring will extend to all who need nursing, for the "protection, promotion, and optimization of health and abilities, prevention of illness and injury, alleviation of suffering through the diagnosis and treatment of human response, and advocacy in the care of individuals, families, communities, and populations."[68]

2. Primacy of the Patient: That the patient's needs and interests supersede those of the institution or the nurse. Conflicts of interest are to be resolved in favor of the patient. The trustworthiness of the nursing profession and its individual members rests upon the primacy of the patient's care, needs, and interests. Professional organizations may seek to benefit nurses but are expected to hold societal and nursing, or patient and nurse, interests in balance: nursing may not gain at the expense of the patient or society.

3. Knowledge, Skill, and Competence: That the profession will ensure the knowledge, skill, and competence of those newly entering practice and those in practice, at every level and in every role. This requires that the profession establish standards for education and practice, oversee education through accreditation, and address error, incompetence, unethical, unprofessional, or impaired practice.

4. Hazardous Service: That members of the profession will provide nursing care under conditions not customarily expected of those outside the profession. This includes exposure to pathogens, contagion, infectious and communicable disease, perseverance under difficult conditions such as weather emergencies and powergrid failures, and caring for patients who are combative or violent.

5. Responsibility and Accountability: That nursing and nurses will be accountable and responsible for practice, transparent when lapses occur, engage in self-regulation and peer-review, and establish and oversee policies for the profession.

6. Progress and Development: That the profession will incorporate knowledge development from the humanities and scientific advances; expand the knowledge base of the profession through theory development, research, scholarship, and innovation; and contribute to the larger sphere of scientific knowledge beyond nursing.

7. Ethical Practice: That the profession will promulgate, affirm, and uphold a code of ethics, to which individual nurses are expected to adhere. That code of ethics will set forth the moral obligations, values, virtues, and ideals of the profession that inform and guide and are incumbent upon the nurse and nursing organizations.

8. Collaboration: That nursing will contribute its distinctive perspective and voice to the wider healthcare conversation, collaborating with other health professions and disciplines to address the health needs of society.

9. Promotion of the Health of the Public: It is expected that nurses will address the problems faced by individual patients including issues of health disparities and that nursing will be involved with and lead in health-related issues important to society. In some instances nursing will be in the vanguard of emerging health-related issues. Nursing will participate in the promulgation of healthcare policy at regional, state, national, and global levels. Protection of the public through advocacy also includes whistleblowing.

Nursing's Expectations of Society within the Social Contract

Contracts are agreements between two parties, thus there are reciprocal obligations or expectations. Just as society has expectations of nursing within the social contract, nursing has expectations of society within that same social contract. Those expectations include the following.

10. Autonomy of Practice: That society will authorize nursing to practice within its scope and standards in identifying and addressing the health needs of the patient, whether individual, family, community, or the nation. This also includes the autonomy to educate its practitioners. Social trust is an aspect of autonomy of practice; nursing expects social trust.

11. Self-governance: That society will extend the authority to professional self-regulation of practice in accord with state nurse practice acts (NPAs). This includes setting the nursing profession's priorities for the health of the nation; establishing scope, standards, and certification processes; interacting with international health-related bodies; and accrediting nursing schools and programs.

12. **Title and Practice Protection:** That society will promulgate law that governs nursing including maintaining and administering licensing examinations, and granting licensure that is mandatory, not permissive. Society will also protect the title "Registered Nurse," and prevent encroachment upon nursing practice.

13. **Respect and Just Remuneration:** That society will accord the nursing profession respect, support for the profession in research and education funding, and a voice at the table. Society will support claims to a just wage and humane work conditions for nurses.

14. **Freedom to Practice:** That nurses will have the authority and freedom to practice nursing to the full extent of their education and preparation, including expanded roles and innovative venues, consistent with state NPAs. That restraints upon nursing that restrict its legitimate practice will be removed.

15. **Workforce Sustainability:** That society will develop, implement, and support a strategic plan to address workforce shortages, workforce sustainability, and workforce capacity. This includes expanding access to nursing education and creating structures for upward educational mobility.

16. **Protection in Hazardous Service:** That society will provide legislative and other means to require organizations to minimize risk to nurses in the face of hazardous service. Nurses are expected to engage in service that carries risks to health above what is expected of the general public.

These 16 elements together constitute the social contract between nursing and society. These categories have some overlap, and could be reconfigured and titled differently, but this nonetheless remains the content of the social contract. An extended discussion of the social contract itself would necessitate taking each of these 16 elements and expanding them. We will not pause to do that here, but instead will continue to explore the essential conceptual building blocks that lay the foundation for understanding the relationship between nursing and society.

Nursing's Social Policy Statement turns its attention to a number of these elements of the social contract. First, it identifies the functions of ANA as "the professional organization that performs an essential function in articulating, maintaining, and strengthening the social contract that exists between nursing and society, upon which the authority to practice nursing is based."[69] Of the 16 elements of nursing's social contract, *Nursing's Social Policy Statement* very briefly addresses ethical practice, collaboration, the knowledge base of practice, and autonomy of practice. Its greatest attention is given to the scope of nursing practice, standards of practice, and the regulation of professional nursing. It does not address all of the elements of nursing's social contract.

Society has a need for caring activity in health and illness; it authorizes a social group called *nursing* to meet that need. In doing so, it accords nursing specific privileges and expectations within the social contract. The broad obligations of nursing are articulated in ANA's definition of nursing as "the protection, promotion, and optimization of health and abilities, prevention of illness and injury, alleviation of suffering through the diagnosis and treatment of human response, and advocacy in the care of individuals, families, communities, and populations."[70]

Nursing engages in an extraordinary range of activities to live out these defining attributes—and in doing so, to meet the needs of society.

Gedankenexperimente: Some Thought Experiments for Nurses about Social Contract Theory

The practical applicability of social contract theory is not immediately evident. As an abstract conceptualization, it is not directly applicable to nursing practice (or to other professional disciplinary practices other than, say, philosophy or the history of ideas); yet it has implications for nursing that are profound both for the ways in which we think about nursing, and for the practice of nursing in terms of its engagement with society. It has particular relevance to nursing's concern for the social causes of health disparities. Social contract theory raises a number of crucial philosophical, theoretical, and ethical questions for nursing that make useful thought experiments both for self-reflection and to clarify how larger conceptual schemata might interact with nursing theory or practice. For example:

- What is nursing's view of person (and human nature), health, society, and nursing (the metaparadigm concepts) versus the understanding of these concepts within social contract theory?

- Does one's view of human nature affect how one conceives of sickness, health, or suffering?

- Is social contract theory an adequate explanation of nursing's relationship to society?

- What dimensions of social contract theory might be troubling for nursing?

- As a discipline that engages in caring practices, does nursing socially devalue its own practices?

- Does social contract afford nursing, as a female-dominated profession, a place at the table?

- Is the social status or social location of nursing affected by social contractarianism?

- Of those whom nursing serves, who is left out of the social contract and how?

- Is the contractarian emphasis on individuality, rationality, self-determination, and the protection of property inimical to nursing's emphasis on caring?

- Is the Kantian autonomy and rationality ultimately compatible with nursing ethics?

- Following Tronto, how might the social contract/politics be changed to incorporate and value caring, an ethic of care, and caring practices?

- Is there a global social contract and, if so, what are its parameters, both in general and specifically for health professions, health professional education, and global health?

- Does social contract have the best fit as a description of nursing's relationship with society?

- Are there alternative theoretical structures for the social and political relationship of professions (nursing) to society that more fully incorporate nursing values?

- Given that social contracts evolve and differ both over time and across nations and cultures, is there an elemental or basic social contract that might include all nurses?

It is important to think about questions such as these in order to formulate a clear and thoughtful perspective on the place of nursing in society and any tensions that may exist between prevailing social contractual views of nursing and the values and ideals that nursing holds dear.

ENDNOTES

All URLs provided are accurate as of May 29, 2015.

1. American Nurses Association (ANA), *Nursing's Social Policy Statement: The Essence of the Profession* (Silver Spring, MD: ANA, 2010).

2. American Nurses Association (ANA), *Nursing: Scope and Standards of Practice* (Silver Spring, MD: ANA, 2010).

3. American Nurses Association (ANA), *Code of Ethics for Nurses with Interpretive Statements* (Silver Spring, MD: ANA, 2015).

4. Note that many of these ancient or early works are in the public domain and are readily available, gratis, in full-text online.

5. Plato *Crito*, Public Domain Book. http://classics.mit.edu/Plato/crito.html.

6. Richard Kraut, *Socrates and the State* (Princeton, New Jersey: Princeton University, 1984).

7. Plato, *Republic*, trans. Robin Waterfield (New York: Oxford University Press, 1993).

8. Epicurus, *Principle Doctrines*, trans. Robert Drew Hicks (Internet Classics Online, 2009).

9. *See also*: http://classics.mit.edu/Epicurus/princdoc.html.

10. Thomas Hobbes, *Leviathan*, ed. Richard Tuck, Cambridge Texts in the History of Political Thought (Cambridge, UK: Cambridge University Press, 1992). *See also:* Thomas Hobbes, *The Leviathan* (Corvallis, OR: Oregon State University, n.d.) http://oregonstate.edu/instruct/phl302/texts/hobbes/leviathan-contents.html.

11. Hobbes, *Leviathan* (1990), 70. Spellings have been modernized.

12. Ibid.

13. Ibid., 80.

14. Ibid.

15. John Locke, *Two Treatises of Government*, ed. Peter Laslett, Cambridge Texts in the History of Political Thought (Cambridge, UK: Cambridge University Press, 1988).

16. Ibid., 79.

17. Ibid., 87.

18. Ibid.

19. Ibid., 79.

20. 20 Ibid.

21. Jean-Jacques Rousseau, *The Basic Political Writings*, ed. and trans. Donald A. Cress, 2nd ed. (Indianapolis: Hackett Publishing, 2011).

22. Ibid., 72.

23. Ibid., 77.

24. Ibid., 87.

25. Ibid., 164.

26. Ibid., 163.

27 J. Maxwell, personal correspondence with the author (May 26, 2015).

28 Bryan Garner, ed., *Black's Law Dictionary*, 10th ed. (Eagan, MN: Thomson West, 2014) 736–37.

29 United States Constitution, Preamble. Full U.S. Constitution available at http://www.archives.gov/exhibits/charters/constitution_transcript.html.

30 John Rawls, *A Theory of Justice* (Cambridge, MA: Harvard/Belknap Press, 1972).

31 Ibid., 3.

32 Ibid., 14–15.

33 Ibid., 123.

34 Ibid., 44, 78.

35 Ibid., 75.

36 Ibid., 87.

37 Sheryl Reimer-Kirkham, "Nursing Research on Religion and Spirituality through a Social Justice Lens," *Advances in Nursing Science* 37, no. 3 (2014): 249–57. See also: Jamie Rogers and Ursula Kelly, "Feminist Intersectionality: Bringing Social Justice to Health Disparities Research," *Nursing Ethics* 18, no. 3 (2011): 397–407; and Kimberly van Herk, Dawn Smith, and Caroline Andrew, "Examining Our Privileges and Oppressions: Incorporating an Intersectionality Paradigm into Nursing," *Nursing Inquiry* 18, no. 1 (2011): 29–39.

38 Kimberlé Crenshaw, "Demarginalization of the Intersection of Race and Sex: A Black Feminist Critique of Antidiscrimination Doctrine, Feminist Theory and Antiracist Politics," University of Chicago Legal Forum, 140 (1989). *See also:* 139–67; Crenshaw, "Intersectionality: The Double Bind of Race and Gender," *Perspectives*, Spring 2004: 2; and Ashley Crossman, "Critical Theory: An Overview," About.com, n.d., http://sociology.about.com/od/Sociological-Theory/a/Critical-Theory.htm.

39 Carole Pateman, *The Sexual Contract* (Cambridge, UK: Polity Press, 1988). *See also*: Pateman, "God Hath Ordained to Man a Helper": Hobbes, Patriarchy and Conjugal Rights," *British Journal of Political Science* 19, no. 4 (October 1989): 445–63; Pateman, *The Problem of Political Obligation: A Critique of Liberal Theory* (Cambridge, UK: Polity Press, 1985); and Pateman, *Participation and Democratic Theory* (Cambridge, UK: Cambridge University Press, 1970).

40 Eva Kittay, Bruce Jennings, and Angela Wasunna, "Dependency, Difference and the Global Ethic of Longterm Care," *Journal of Political Philosophy* 13, no. 4 (2005): 443–69. *See also:* Eva Kittay and Ellen Feder, ed., *The Subject of Care: Feminist Perspectives on Dependency* (Lanham, MD: Rowman & Littlefield, 2002).

41 Annette C. Baier, *Moral Prejudices: Essays on Ethics*, (Cambridge, MA: Harvard University Press, 1995).

42 Jean Hampton, *Hobbes and the Social Contract Tradition* (Cambridge, UK: Cambridge University Press, 1988). *See also:* Hampton, "Two Faces of Contractarian Thought," in *Contractarianism and Rational Choice; Essays on David Gauthier's Morals by Agreement*, ed. Peter Vallentyne (Cambridge, UK: Cambridge University Press, 1991), 31–55; and Hampton, "Feminist Contractarianism," in *A Mind of One's Own: Feminist Essays on Reason and Objectivity*, ed. Louise M. Antony and Charlotte E. Witt, 2nd ed. (Boulder, CO: Westview, 2002), 337–68.

43 Jean B. Elshtain, *Public Man, Private Woman* (Princeton, NJ: Princeton University Press, 1981).

44 Virginia Held, "Noncontractual Society: A Feminist View," in *Science, Morality and Feminist Theory*, ed. M. P. Hanen and K. Nielson, *Canadian Journal of Philosophy* Supplement (Calgary, CA: University of Calgary Press, 1987), 111–37.

45 Susan M. Okin, *Justice, Gender and the Family* (New York: Basic Books, 1989).

46 Mari J. Matsuda, "Liberal Jurisprudence and Abstracted Visions of Human Nature: A Feminist Critique of Rawls' Theory of Justice," *New Mexico Law Review* 16, no. 3 (Fall 1986): 613–30. *See also:* David Boucher and Paul Kelly, "The Social Contract and Its Critics: An Overview," in *The Social Contract from Hobbes to Rawls*, ed. D. Boucher and P. Kelly (London: Routledge, 1994), 1–34; Diane Coole, "Women, Gender and Contract: Feminist Interpretations," in Boucher and Kelly, *Social Contract*, 191–210; Carol Gilligan, *In a Different Voice: Psychological Theory and Women's Development* (Cambridge, MA: Harvard University Press, 1982); Crawford B. Macpherson, *The Political Theory of Possessive Individualism: Hobbes to Locke* (Oxford, UK: Oxford University Press, 1962); John S. Mill, *The Subjection of Women*, in *On Liberty and Other Essays*, ed. John Gray (Oxford, UK: Oxford University Press, 1998) 469–582; and Ruth Sample, "Why Feminist Contractarianism?" *Journal of Social Philosophy* 33, no. 2 (2002): 257–81.

47 Pateman, *Sexual Contract*, x.

48 Ibid., 6.

49 Ibid., 2.

50 Ibid., 3.

51 Kittay, Jennings, and Wasunna, "Longterm Care," 443.

52 Rhacel Parreñas and Eileen Boris, *Intimate Labors: Cultures, Technologies, and the Politics of Care* (Stanford, CA: Stanford University Press, 2010).

53 Joan Tronto, *Moral Boundaries: A Political Argument for an Ethic of Care* (New York: Routledge, 1993), 54.

54 Ibid., 55–56.

55 Held, "Noncontractual Society," 194–95.

56 Tronto, *Moral Boundaries*, 54.

57 Charles W. Mills, *The Racial Contract*, (Ithaca, NY: Cornell University Press, 2014), 3.

58 Ibid., 4.

59 Anita Silvers and Leslie Francis, "Justice through Trust: Disability and the 'Outlier Problem' in Social Contract Theory," *Ethics* 116, no. 1 (October 2005): 40–41.

[60] Kittay, Jennings, Wasunna, "Longterm Care," 445.

[61] Gorik Ooms et al., "A Global Social Contract to Reduce Maternal Mortality: The Human Rights Arguments and the Case of Uganda," *Reproductive Health Matters* 21, no. 42 (2013): 129–38.

[62] Thomas Donaldson and Thomas Dunfee, "Toward a Unified Conception of Business Ethics: Integrative Social Contracts Theory," *Academy of Management Review* 19, no. 2 (1994) 252–84.

[63] American Medical Association, *Code of Medical Ethics of the American Medical Association* (Chicago: American Medical Association, 1847), 105.

[64] Matthew K. Wynia. "The Short History and Tenuous Future of Medical Professionalism: The Erosion of Medicine's Social Contract," Perspectives in Biology and Medicine, 51, no. 4 (Autumn 2008): 567.

[65] Richard Cruess and Sylvia Cruess, "Expectations and Obligations: Professionalism and Medicine's Social Contract with Society," *Perspectives in Biology and Medicine* 51, no. 4 (Autumn 2008): 583.

[66] Ibid., 586.

[67] "Public Ranks Nurses as Most Honest, Ethical Profession for 13th Straight Year (12/18/14)," NursingWorld.org, 2014, http://nursingworld.org/Nurses-MostHonestEthicalProfession.

[68] "What is nursing?" NursingWorld.org, http://www.nursingworld.org/EspeciallyForYou/What-is-Nursing.

[69] ANA, *Nursing's Social Policy Statement*, 6.

[70] Ibid.

[71] Max Horkheimer, *Critical Theory* (New York: Seabury Press, 1972) 246.

Chapter 2.
Nursing as Profession
A Pugilistic Journey

In Chapter 1, we examined the theories of social contract and their critiques. That chapter looked at social contracts in relation to professions, specifically the professions of medicine and nursing. Since the focus of the social contract is its relationship with professions, this chapter turns to the topic of professions and asks "What is a profession?" We will need to address the more basic concepts of occupation, vocation, and calling, as well as the historic emergence of professions before actually turning to how professions are defined or identified. There are a number of approaches to identifying or defining professions and we will look at six. The chapter will close with a discussion of the forms of control of occupational labor, profession being one form of occupational control, and perspectives on the role of professions in society.

Nursing as an Occupation, Vocation, Calling, and Profession

Nursing's history has been something of a roller-coaster ride. In the West, its early days as an occupation were most frequently associated with nursing religious orders. It was considered a "high calling" to care for the sick. In England, hospitals were established in the 1100s (St. Bartholomew's, 1123) and 1200s, and staffed by religious nursing orders. Religious orders, too, suffered their own woes with the dissolution of the monasteries in 1539.[1] At that point, religious support for hospitals ended and care of the sick, "no longer transformed by the devotion of religious enthusiasm, appeared a sordid duty, only fit for the lowest class in the community."[2] Into the 1800s, nursing remained in bad straights, as can be seen by Charles Dickens's infamous caricature of a nurse, Sarah "Sairy" Gamp in his picaresque novel *The Life and Adventures of Martin Chuzzlewit* (1843). Mrs. Gamp is a drunken, dissolute, dissipated, disgusting, opportunistic, and incompetent nurse and midwife. Elizabeth Fry, Florence Nightingale, and others brought about a drastic reform in nursing education and practice. English authors Carr-Saunders and Wilson, early sociologists of professions, write this about nursing:

The ancient vocation of nursing has passed through vicissitudes without parallel in any other vocation which comes under review [in this book]. This may be traced to the fact that until recently the only nursing worthy of the name was inspired by religious or at least philanthropic motives. Nurses were 'called' to a life devoted to the alleviation of suffering, and when the 'call' was not given or not heard the task was left undone or was abandoned to persons to whom the honorable title of nurse was not appropriate.[3]

Carr-Saunders and Wilson's book *The Professions* (1933) is one of the earliest thorough works on professions and professionalism. In their brief treatment of nursing, surprising for its inclusion at all, they are warmly sympathetic toward nursing. After discussing the development and transformation of nursing in Britain, they write that

nursing has thus undergone a transformation. …The dignity of the vocation has been enhanced…all working towards the conception of the building up of a skilled and responsible vocation. …Until lately, however, the nurse worked under the direction of the doctor, and there was little element of co-operation. While the nurse must continue to work under direction, the tendency is towards co-operation which is made possible by the higher training…the vocation of nursing has become professionalized. …We must look for the explanation…in the fact that a skilled and dignified profession may also be in [Nightingale's] sense a 'calling.'[4]

Nursing is an occupation, vocation, calling, and profession. To understand nursing's journey, hard-fought, to the standing of a profession, it is necessary to unpack these terms.

THINKING ABOUT HENRY, WHO WANTS A SON…

Who knew that Henry VIII's determination to produce a male heir would affect nursing history? English school children learn the rhyme to remember the fate of Henry's wives: "Divorced, Beheaded, Died; Divorced, Beheaded, Survived." England was Catholic and Henry's wife Catherine of Aragon produced only a daughter, Mary. The Pope would not grant Henry a divorce so that he could marry another in an attempt to produce a male heir, so Henry severed the church relationship with Rome and created the Church of England. The Catholic monasteries were wealthy and powerful. By the dissolution of the monasteries Henry would, and did, gain money, lands, more power and at the same time could remove a large source of papist influence. The dissolution of the monasteries, which began in 1536, ended the Roman Catholic religious orders, including the religious nursing orders, and support for religious hospitals. Carr writes that "in England, nursing was no longer a religious vocation and, being poorly paid, it came to be regarded as menial service and attracted only paupers, drunken [sic] and the inefficient." (Carr, 1915; p. 187.) Where is Florence Nightingale when we need her? Oh, 284 years away.

Occupation and Vocation, Livelihood and Calling
Occupation

Surnames make a fascinating and complex study. They take different structures, order, and modes of acquisition in different languages and cultures. In a number of languages they indicate lineage through a patronymic formed from the father's name; for example, in Welsh, John, son of Owen would be John ap Owen (later John Bowen), Richard ap Evan (becoming Bevan), or William ap David (becoming William Davies or Davis). In Scandinavian languages, the construction Thorsen indicates a son of Thor, or Knuteson a son of Knute; in Spanish, Fernandez would be a son of Fernando, or Rodrigues, a son of Rodrigo. In Icelandic, Jóhanna Sigurðardóttir is Jóhanna, daughter of Sigurð[ur], and in Russian, Svetlana Ivanovna is Svetlana, daughter of Ivan. Other surnames are descriptive of the person, such as Tom Swift, William Lovejoy, or Samuel Long (indicating tall). The names Franklin and Fry refer to one who is free-born. Some surnames are locative, indicating the place of origin of the person, such as Meadows, Wood, Lane, and Fields. Still others, and more to the point here, were occupational surnames such as Fletcher (maker of arrow feathers), Fowler (bird keeper), Tinker (itinerant mender of metal utensils), Taylor, Saylor, Cooper (barrel maker), Fuller (one who fulls cloth), Chandler (candlemaker), and Wainwright (wagon builder). Is there a surname indicating a nurse? The French surname Nurse

> is an occupational name for a wet nurse or foster mother, deriving from the Old French "nurice, norrice". ...Early examples of the surname include: Matilda Nutrix and Maria le Noreyse (Cambridgeshire, 1273); Alice la Norisse and Agnes le Norice... dated 1310 to 1337; and Joan Nurys, recorded with Magota Nuris in the 1379 Poll Tax Returns of Yorkshire. Recordings of the surname from London Church Registers include: ...Margery Nourse... and the christening of Elizabeth, daughter of Peter Nurse...1601. An early settler in the New World was Robert Nurse. ...A Coat of Arms [was] granted to the Nurse family of England. ...The first recorded spelling of the family name is shown to be that of Roberta la Norice, which was dated 1273, in the "Hundred Rolls of Bedfordshire", during the reign of King Edward 1...1272–1307.[5]

Occupational surnames once indicated the type of work that one could do, and more often indicated the livelihood that occupied one's time in earning a living. Surnames can seem amusing but, historically speaking, they signal a coalescing public recognition of divisions of labor that had emerged as specific—and paid—occupations. From the early 1300s onward, then, the occupation of nurse finds its way into surnames. In the past, there might have been only one tanner, smith, sawyer, and cooper in a town, but as population density increased, so did the number of people involved in the same occupation.

Eventually members of an occupation living in close proximity to one another would form an associative group such as a guild, confraternity, secret society, or association. These were largely (though not exclusively) men's groups, as the majority of women did not work outside the home and caring functions such as nursing remained "hidden" within homes. Guilds were of two types—artisans and craftsmen or merchants—and they controlled the exercise of their respective trades within a specific town or city. Rousseau was a strong critic of the guild system as he supported *laissez-faire* market system. Guilds failed with the advent of industrialization and modernization and the advent of free-trade laws. Safartti Larson believes that modern medicine's professional association initially had a guild-like structure.[6] However, these groups of workers did not yet constitute professions as we understand professions today, though they could be vocations.

Vocation and Calling

The term *vocation* comes from the Latin *vocatio*, a call or summons. Historically it has been a reference to a divine calling to serve God, the Church, or humanity with the specific abilities that one has been given. Thomas Aquinas (1225–1274) saw vocation as a social office that is only a vocation insofar as it serves the common good and does not harm. He created a hierarchy of vocations including judges, military, farmers, artisans, and merchants. He ranked farmers highest and merchants lowest, though all secular vocations were lower than explicitly religious vocations.[7] In the Protestant Reformation, vocation included all or any occupational labor that was specifically secular in nature, as long as the individual was called to the exercise of that specific occupation.[8] The Reformers refuted any notion of a hierarchy of occupational labor. Reformer John Calvin's (1509–1564) vocational idea was that "there would be no employment so mean and sordid (provided we follow our vocation) as not to appear truly respectable, and be deemed highly important in the sight of God."[9] So, whether lofty or humble, philosopher or chimney sweep, all occupations were equally worthy. It must be noted that some current usages of *vocation*, as in *vocational education*, signify not a calling, but a form of education for manual trades such as automobile repair, welding, and tool and die makers. Vocation is not used in that sense in this book.

But vocation is an odd term. Is nursing a vocation? For those in nursing who are not called to nursing the answer is no. Some enter "nursing" for economic reasons, some out of a sense of obligation, or family pressure. There are any number of reasons one might enter nursing without being called. But doing so turns nursing work into toil or a job and nursing does not become a resident part of the person's identity. For those who are called to nursing, it is a vocation, it is something much more than a job, it becomes an abiding part of one's identity. This is the nurse who does not simply *do* nursing; this is the nurse who *is* a nurse: it is a matter of being over doing. At some point an occupation may develop into a profession. From the earliest moments of the rise of modern nursing, its leaders understood nursing to be a true profession.

Nightingale: Called by God but a Non-Religious Nursing School

The notion of nursing as a vocation or calling, (the terms are used interchangeably), persists in the nursing literature. Florence Nightingale (1820–1910) felt herself called by God, and more specifically called to nursing as service. However, she also came to regard nursing itself as a calling and wrote to probationers (early nursing students) and nurses that "nursing is said, most truly said, to be a high calling, an honorable calling."[10] Nightingale's life

> was lived out in service to God through her call to nursing and her embrace of nursing as a high calling in itself. As she moved into nursing education she demanded a rigorous education for women who would become nurses. Surprisingly, however, she sought a thoroughly secularized nursing education.[11]

Nightingale scholar Lynn Macdonald, who has compiled the complete works of Nightingale, writes:

> The exacting workload, character, and devotion long required of the nurse go back to Nightingale's conceptualization of nursing as a religious *calling*, a calling to patient care and health promotion. She abhorred nurses acting as missionaries to save the souls of the sick or dying, which prompted her to insist that her training school for nurses be non-sectarian.[12]

Nightingale wanted to accept students into her school independent of their religious commitment. Even so, while the school was to be non-sectarian, it was nevertheless Christian. Again McDonald writes,

> Nightingale wanted nurses to be ordinary women, not nuns, and the profession to be open to all without any religious test. But her letters to nurses and nursing students are full of religious material, advice and prayers, for she believed that nurses needed ongoing spiritual nourishment. …While Nightingale insisted that her training school be non-sectarian, accepting students on the basis of merit regardless

of religion, there was a significant Christian (indeed Church of England) element in the daily routine.[13]

So nursing education was secularized yet retained a strong concept of vocation as a call from God. Eventually the concept would become neutral so that it could be understood in either secular or religious terms as a vocation to which one was committed, not to *do* nursing, but to *be* a nurse. Nursing, then, was not a job or occupation, it was more than that; it was a calling and a profession in the sense of what one professes so that it was inextricably tied to one's identity and way of being in the world.

Did Nightingale regard nursing as both a vocation and a profession? Yes… and no. When Nightingale entered nursing she undertook to elevate it from a less than reputable activity to an educated, trained, prepared, scientific, and cultivated profession.[14] After returning from her work in Crimea and establishing Nightingale model schools of nursing she did in fact move nursing into a new social, educational, and occupational status. She did, however, live in that uneasy eschatological tension of something that is now, but is also yet to come. Yes, nursing was a calling or vocation, but it was also a nascent profession, beginning its growth and development under her watchful eye—and the extensive labors of her quill.

The Emergence of Professions

In the High Middle Ages, the late 11th through the 13th centuries, the first European universities were established for the study of theology, law, and medicine.[15] For centuries these three disciplines would remain the only recognized professions. The noted essayist Joseph Addison (1672–1719) referred to them as "the three great professions divinity, law and physic."[16] These professions were referred to as *learnéd professions*, as entry into practice required a university education. A Bachelor of Arts was earned in the third or fourth year on the way to a Master of Arts. Students were required to become accomplished in seven liberal arts: arithmetic, geometry, astronomy, music theory, grammar, logic, and rhetoric, which was foundational learning. After completion of the Master of Arts, the student could then enter one of the higher faculties to study law, medicine, or theology. Of the three learned professions, theology remained the most prestigious for centuries;[17] it was the first profession and remained the only profession until joined by medicine and law, and later architecture, commissioned military service, and possibly teaching.[18] It is important to note here the university education was required of each of the learned professions, and that entry into these professions was built upon a base of both a master's degree and a liberal arts education.

Knowing that there were three groups that were regarded as professions does not answer the question "What is a profession?" Sociologist John Archer Jackson writes

> The main issues which have been debated in the study of professions and professionalization centre around the problems of distinguishing a profession from a non-profession, and of discerning the processes of professionalization. With the former problem, the major task is usually thought to involve the isolation of sets of critical discriminating characteristics or variables. …In contrast, the professionalization approach commonly rests on a set of assumptions, often implicit, about the nature of a profession, while the main emphasis is placed upon the identification of some sort of development sequence.[19]

Like defining *human* so that it encompasses all persons no matter their condition, but without including robots and dolphins, defining *profession* has similar problems of inclusion and exclusion. Distinguishing between profession and craft is one such example. Though there are important outliers on either end, such as Carr-Saunders and Wilson,[20] who wrote from the late 1920s into the 1930s, and Freidson,[21] (a noted sociologist who studied the structure of professions), in the present who writes principally on medicine, the bulk of the writing on the rise and nature of professions takes place in the 1950s through the 1970s. This may be a consequence of the escalation of divisions of labor in society that attend the advance of science and technology. The road to defining profession has been filled with controversy, argument, and a lack of consensus that has been refractory to resolution. As a consequence, there are multiple approaches to how a profession might be defined.

Some Approaches to Defining Profession

Millerson identifies three means of defining professions that remain the major approaches.[22] Cheetham and Chivers add another three approaches, all of

---

THINKING ABOUT GOOD AND EVIL…

Why would an occupational group want society to regard it as a profession? It's not hard to understand why. With the status of profession, occupational groups have social prestige, authority, recognition, and financial reward. All of this gives them power. That power can be used altruistically to benefit society and be a moral force for good, or selfishly to reinforce monopolistic power elites, restrain other groups, garner excessive wealth, exploit those needing their services, and increase political power. It is important to think about how various occupational groups that have gained social power have used that power. Physicians, politicians, entertainers, attorneys, teachers, professors, artists—as groups (not as individuals), how have these occupations used their social power?

---

which are less common.[23] Each of the six approaches is discussed below. The six approaches are as follows:

1. Looking for a set of characteristics or traits associated with professions.

2. Looking for evidence of professionalization (the process through which occupations are said to become professions).

3. Developing a model of professionalism based on certain sociological aspects of professional practice.

4. Adopting a classification system based on socioeconomic factors, e.g., *Standard Occupational Classifications.*

5. Examining the complexity of the competencies involved (which may have some relationship to the level of a qualification, as is the case with the UK National Vocational Qualifications).

6. Following the societal view of which jobs are seen as professions.

The Trait Approach

The first approach has been the one that predominates in the nursing literature in the defense of nursing as a profession. This approach identifies requisite traits or specific attributes of professions by which occupational groups are judged.

Trait definitions abound and form the backbone of many of the discussions of nursing as a profession.[24] They often focus on a core that includes (a) a well-defined body of knowledge; (b) specialized education and expertise based in higher education; (c) provision of a practical service; (d) existence of a professional association; (e) autonomy of practice; (f) profession-determined standards or practice and education; (g) adumbration of a code of ethics; and (h) altruistic motivation.[25] Within a trait definition framework, whether or not an

---

THINKING ABOUT BARBERS, SURGEONS AND DENTISTS...

Professions emerge and develop; they do not spring forth full-grown. Take the case of surgeons. Physicians in ancient Greece were forbidden to do surgery with the sole exception of surgery for renal calculi. Surgery was disdainful and distasteful as an occupation as it engaged in "manualism," the use of the hands rather than the mind. In medieval Europe, barber surgeons were medical practitioners who would extract teeth, perform enemas, sell medicines, do bloodletting, lance cataracts, perform surgery—oh, and cut hair, shave beards, and perform manicures. Barbers had blades and knew how to use them. It is not until the mid-1700s that barbers and surgeons and dentists go their separate ways. (For additional insights along these lines: visit the Londons Science Museum's History of Medicine website: http://www.sciencemuseum.org.uk/broughtto-life.aspx .)

occupational group is to be regarded as a profession depends on its realization of the attributes specified.[26]

Discussions of nursing as a profession have focused on nursing's possession of all of these traits. In recent decades much of this discussion has centered on the possession of a well-defined body of knowledge that is distinctive from that of medicine and, more pointedly, the criterion of autonomy of practice. Much of the discussion of the metaparadigm concepts of nursing, theories of nursing, and nursing diagnoses has been historically important in sharpening the distinction between medicine and nursing, even if that distinction has not been widely known or understood outside of nursing—or by medicine. The continued development of nursing research, that is, nursing science, has pretty much dissolved this discussion: nursing possesses a distinctive body of knowledge. It is the issue of autonomy that has remained a sticking point, though less so in the past 20 years. Cheetham and Chivers, who study professional development in the UK, point out that Freidson

> makes a distinction between professionals and paraprofessionals. He uses the term 'paraprofessional' to describe occupations such as Nursing which, whilst they possess some of the characteristics of the medical profession with which they are closely associated, are nonetheless subordinate to it. In his view, nurses are not full professionals because they, like the military, lack autonomy.[27]

However, in his more recent 2001 work, *Professionalism: The Third Logic*, Freidson writes:

> If one can stretch the method a bit and create an ideal type for an impure or incomplete social form like semi-profession, one might call it an occupation that has gained jurisdiction in a division of labor, as well as a labor market shelter and control over its own training, credentialing, and supervision, but that has not established sufficient cognitive authority to dominate either the division of labor in which its jurisdiction is located or public discourse concerning its work. A crude measure of this weak economic and cultural authority is its relatively low but by no means ignominious social status.[28]

In his evolving schema, nursing has some of the elements of autonomy of practice, but not others. Nursing would remain one of Freidson's semi-professions to the degree that it did not have "cognitive authority to dominate either the division of labor in which its jurisdiction is located or public discourse concerning its work." Nursing, today, does dominate the division of its own labor. Whether it dominates the public discourse concerning its work is an open question, and whether this is a determinative criterion of professionalism is subject to disagreement, particularly with the growth of mediative control of occupational labor (discussed below).

Control of one's work, which Freidson terms *professionalism* (or *autonomy*), is critical to his analysis. He writes:

> Professionalism may be said to exist when an organized occupation gains the power to determine who is qualified to perform a defined set of tasks, to prevent all others from performing that work, and to control the criteria by which to evaluate performance. In the case of professionalism, neither individual buyers of labor in the market nor the managers of bureaucratic firms have the right to themselves choose workers to perform particular tasks or evaluate their work except within the limits specified by the occupation. The organized occupation creates the circumstances under which its members are free of control by those who employ them.[29]

If nursing did not rise to the level of professionalism that Freidson accorded professions in his early writings, it does so now. As to trait definitions of professions generally, there is a tautological problem in trait definitions. The traits are largely derived by identifying existing professions and deriving from them a set of traits that define professions. It becomes tautological because it asserts that "these are the traits of a profession because these are the traits that a profession possesses." Trait approaches assume that there are "true" professions and that they will demonstrate all of the essential core attributes. However, the attributes themselves are often an untidy aggregation of overlapping, arbitrarily chosen, or undifferentiated elements, lacking a unifying theoretical framework that explains their interrelationship. Trait theories tend to empirically generate a definition of a profession and then ascribe to it a normative rather than a descriptive status.[30] Traits, then, become a matter of seeing what one is looking for.

The Professionalization Approach

The second approach posits that there are stages that occupations go through in becoming a profession. This approach is championed by Caplow,[31] Vollmer and Mills,[32] and Wilensky.[33] Wilensky's stages are

1. Start doing full time the thing that needs doing.

2. Establish a training school: if the school does not start in a university it nonetheless develops standards for education, academic degrees, research, and standards.

3. Form a professional association.

4. Political agitation in order to win the support of law for the protection of the job territory and its sustaining code of ethics….

5. Establish a formal code of ethics with rules to eliminate the unqualified and unscrupulous, reduce internal competition, and protect clients.[34]

Wilinsky notes that a number of groups are in the process of professionalizing and that "there are borderline cases such as school-teaching, librarianship, nursing, pharmacy, [and] optometry."[35] The studies he relies upon for this assertion are from the 1950s and do not reflect the situation of any of these occupations today. He, like Freidson and others, regards nursing as "ancillary to medicine."[36] The professionalization model bears the same tautological problem as that of the trait definitions.

The Sociological Approach

This model was advanced by T. H. Marshall[37] and later by Ernest Greenwood. Greenwood describes the sociological approach as

> one that views a profession as an organized group which is constantly interacting with the society that forms its matrix, which performs its social functions through a network of formal and informal relationships, and which creates its own subculture requiring adjustments to it as a prerequisite for career success.[38]

Within its social matrix, those elements of a profession that interact with society are: "(1) systematic theory, (2) authority, (3) community sanction, (4) ethical codes, and (5) a culture."[39] With regard to systematic theory, Greenwood writes that "a profession's underlying body of theory is a system of abstract propositions that describe in general terms the classes of phenomena comprising the profession's focus of interest."[40] The theory is constructed via systematic research. Mastery of this theory requires extensive education as well as both intellectual and practical experience.[41] The profession's authority rests upon extensive education in a specialized knowledge that has *functional specificity*, a concept advanced by Talcott Parsons.[42] Functional specificity means that the professional has authority only within the sphere of the professional's education. Community sanction means that the community confers upon the profession certain powers and privileges that are, at least in part, enforced by the community's coercive power (including legislation, regulation, legal sanctions). He notes confidentiality as a particular and essential privilege.[43] The regulative code of ethics is essential to offsetting the monopoly of practice that a profession enjoys, and prevents abuses and runaway self-interest: "The ethics governing colleague relationships demand behavior that is co-operative, equalitarian, and supportive."[44] Professional culture entails the existence of three types of organizations: those through which a profession performs service (e.g., firms, agencies, institutions), those that supply practitioners and support knowledge development (e.g., universities), and those that promote the aims and interests of the group (e.g., professional associations). However, beyond organizations, "the culture of a profession consists of its values, norms, and symbols."[45] The values relate to what the profession holds to be the essential service it provides to society. The norms relate to the profession's behavioral guides within social situations. The symbols are meaning bearing and include garb, insignias, history, narrative, historical figures, and more. Greenwood goes on to say that "our discussion of the professional culture would be incomplete without brief mention of one of its central concepts, the *career* concept. ...A career is essentially a calling, a life devoted to 'good works.' Professional work is never viewed solely as a means to an end; it is the end itself."[46]

Socioeconomic Classification Systems Approach

The socioeconomic classification systems, the fourth approach, is to accept as professions those occupational groups regarded as such in official government publications—such as the U.S. government's *Standard Occupational Classification*,[47] and *Handbook of Occupational Groups and Families*,[48] the International Standard Classification of Occupations (ISCO),[49] the European communities Recognition of Professional Qualifications: General Medical (UK),[50] the French classification by the Unions de Recouvrement des Cotisations de Sécurité Sociale et d'Allocations Familiales, (the Organizations for the Payment of Social Security and Family Benefit Contributions), and a range of national and international classification systems. The French Social Security system divides occupations into four categories: artisan, industriel, commerçant (business), and professions libérals (professions). The US document divides the classifications into major categories; category 29-0000 is "Healthcare Practitioners and Technical Occupations." Here, nurses are categorized as "29-1000 Health diagnosing and treating practitioners." The occupational description is:

> Assess patient health problems and needs, develop and implement nursing care plans, and maintain medical records. Administer nursing care to ill, injured, convalescent, or disabled patients. May advise patients on health maintenance and disease prevention or provide case management. Licensing or registration required. Includes Clinical Nurse Specialists. Excludes "Nurse Anesthetists" (29-1151), "Nurse Midwives" (29-1161), and "Nurse Practitioners" (29-1171).[51]

Note that, unlike the international documents, the U.S. classifications do not designate which groups are or are not professions. Some of these documents are concerned chiefly for the reciprocity of credentials across nations. All of these documents classify, at least in part, jobs by skill level, educational requirements, and the nature of the work that is done. In the international documents, nursing is not uniformly situated within professions; the ISCO approach places nurses in the associate professionals category.[52]

It is important to make note of several facts. First, even in the United States, nursing has multiple entry points, some of which do not require advanced degrees characteristic of the learned or liberal professions, or those occupational groups regarded as professions. More importantly, in terms of international classifications, the level of nursing education and practice globally is dramatically uneven (though improving). Thus, if nursing easily rises to the level of profession in one nation, it may well be semi-skilled, low-education labor in another; these classifications give one classification that covers the entire range of global practice. Cheetham and Chivers rightly note the level of "subjectivity and cultural bias" that enters even these classifications but fail to note that the classifications amortization the education requirements, entry points, practice scope and standards across nations.[53] These classifications are descriptive, not normative, and are not useful for determining what is or is not a profession—they only take account descriptively of how the occupations are regarded in different nations.

This category might also include the U.S. Census categories; Freidson rejects the census categories as an adequate basis for determining occupations that are professions. He writes that

> official classificatory schemes are no less subject to social influences than are others—indeed, they may be more subject to them than many others. …The categories are inevitably a partial function of the political processes they serve. Given the fact that official classification as a profession can confer at least symbolic and sometimes real economic benefits on members of an occupation, it is not surprising that active political lobbying may have as much to do with the inclusion of an occupation in the professional category as do the objective educational qualifications of its members. Airline pilots and nurses, neither of whom are required to have college training, lobbied for the elimination of the semiprofessional category in which they were both classified in the 1940 census so that they would be classified in the professional category subsequently. The census categories must be seen as a complex and analytically heterogeneous product of historical interplay among a variety of political, economic, and administrative forces.[54]

We will need to return to the issue of the social construction of categories when we examine the societal view below.

The Complexity of the Competencies Method

In this fifth approach, the level of skill of the occupation's knowledge and practice is assessed and a hierarchy is constructed. There is a hint of this approach in the U.S. *Standard Occupational Classification* noted above. Cheetham and Chivers comment that

> despite their air of rationality. ...a subjective judgement still has to be made as to which level is appropriate for a particular occupation. ...In some cases, decisions may be coloured by political and pragmatic considerations. The approach may therefore be just as likely as any other to suffer from selectivity, tautology and subjectivity.[55]

The approach is used in the United Kingdom, where occupations are ranked as higher-level occupations and lower-level occupations, not using the term professions. The National Vocational Qualification (NVQ) ranks occupations based on the National Occupational Standards that describe occupational competencies.[56] There is an analogous European qualification framework. Because the NVQ is so tightly related to and based on the UK educational system, it is not generalizable to the United States.

The Societal View Approach

The sixth approach, the societal view, is fraught with problems, chiefly that of the social construction of categories based on cultural and social bias. Early professions in the 18th and 19th centuries were dominated by sons of the landed gentry. Land ownership conferred the wealth necessary to secure an education into an occupation suitable for a gentleman, that is, one free of "manualism."[57] Thus, early professions were associated with a particular race, gender, and class, specifically white, male, gentlemen of the aristocracy. As occupations increasingly developed and differentiated it was to their advantage to be regarded as a profession for the social and economic benefit that accrued to professions. Cheetham and Chivers, however, note the social bias in the designation of an occupation as a profession:

> Despite the various rational attempts to find a suitable definition, the classification of particular jobs as professions...may be more of a social than a technical judgement. Society itself seems to have well entrenched views on the status of various occupations. These may cause some to be accepted as professions while others are seen simply as jobs.[58]

The societal view approach, then, is problematic in that it is little more than a reflection of the social biases of the dominant power groups of a society.

Nursing and the Societal View Approach

This approach is particularly important with regard to nursing and teaching (especially elementary and middle school education) as occupational groups that are both female-dominant and, to some extent, share in the same assessment or if not, perhaps, mal-assessment. Again, Cheetham and Chivers note that

> there is of course a difference between the legitimisation of professional authority and the recognition by society of a particular occupation as a profession. The latter may be influenced as much by the political strength of particular occupations, as their contribution to the health and well being of society. It may also be linked to the perceived class position of typical members of society. Such perceptions may have strong roots in the past when entry into the traditional (and only) professions was restricted to people (usually men) from the upper classes. Thus, it can be argued, it was not so much the profession itself, or even its utility to society which conferred status, but rather its association with people who already had status as a result of their birth. ...Society's way of defining professions is likely to be unreliable, and even arbitrary.[59]

Culturally and societally defined social roles and the social location of women have profoundly affected the societal assessment of nursing. The "handmaiden to the physician" or "the physician's hand" (however accurate or inaccurate those models may be) will never be regarded as professional. Even the nurse–scientist might not be regarded as professional where and when cultural or societal biases prevail. Melosh advances a fairly grim prospect for nursing. Writing in 1982, she writes that the stature of medicine as a profession is, in part, predicated upon the continued subordination of nursing:[60]

> Professions are not just special organizations of work but rather particular expressions and vehicles of dominant class and culture. ...Because women are the "second sex," I would argue, there can be no women's profession. ...With few exceptions, white men from upper middle-class backgrounds fill the professions. Within the existing division of labor, nursing is not a profession, because nurses' autonomy is constrained by medicine's professional dominance. In broader cultural terms, nursing by definition cannot be a profession because most nurses are women.[61]

While its status as a historically female-dominated occupation is something nursing shares with elementary teaching and secretary work, its educational structure has differed. Nursing students were generally required to live in hospital residences, which gave nursing its own occupational culture, one that emphasized a particular value structure that included virtue, service, altruism, selflessness, and devotion to the patient, in addition to scientific knowledge and clinical skill.

Nursing remains in a socially disadvantaged position on more than one count. As Melosh and many others have noted, issues of gender and the relationship with medicine, to which might be added issues of race and class, have served to disadvantage nursing. Nursing began with a two-class system within the Nightingale construct. "The Nightingale reforms had intended to make nursing attractive to upper-class women with good preparatory education in addition to the goals of better training and control over the many lower-class recruits."[62] Since early nursing largely took place in the home, it would be necessary for nurses to be of "good character" in order for those who could afford to pay for nursing services to feel comfortable having nurses in their home. Leaders of nursing, in its early modern years in the United States, were white upper-class women. The two-class system of nursing persists in the educational divide between junior/community college (Associate Degree) and college/university (BS, MS, PhD) nurses.[63] In addition, as of 2013, the nursing workforce was 83% white/Caucasian, 90.4% female, and only 12.3% of nursing faculty came from minority backgrounds.[64] Issues of gender, race and class not only surround nursing but affect it from within.

However, both elementary teaching's and nursing's involvement with care work serve to further disadvantage both occupations—to a large extent through the devaluing of care by those outside either profession. The effects on nursing are distinctive:

> The devaluing of care is important as it affects nursing within the institutions and agencies that employ it. However, the devaluing of care is important in the larger global context. …An important body of literature has developed on the devaluation of care as *intimate labor*. Intimate labor is largely behind the scenes labor that is not seen as having the same economic value as, for instance, the fees for nursing care that are folded into a room charge. Nursing falls at the high end of the continuum of intimate labor while housekeeping and childcare fall at the lower end. The concerns of this body of literature are that care is socially and economically devalued. Parreñas and Boris write that "intimate labor emerges as a mechanism that maintains and reflects socioeconomic inequalities." [65] What is important here is that care activities (including nursing care) as

forms of intimate labors are tied to economic structures that perpetuate inequality and support a wide range of unjust structures.[66]

In his 1970 analysis of elementary teaching, Leggatt applies his observations
to both teaching and nursing. He writes that

> the [teaching] occupation can be undertaken by those with the low
> career commitment characteristic of women who wish to raise a
> family at some point in their lives. Today almost all women work
> but only a minority have long-range occupational commitments. Its
> lack of a specialized and rapidly changing knowledge base makes a
> period of absence from practice—even of sufficient length to allow
> the raising of a family—quite manageable for a teacher, without the
> need of a period of re-training.[67]

He writes that teaching "calls upon nurturant skills, and an holistic approach
towards other people that is more culturally developed among women." He
notes the social conditioning of nurturant behavior but then proceeds to write
that "[t]he stereotype of teaching as a women's occupation is, then, founded
in empirical fact in two respects; it is an occupation with a predominance of
women members and it involves work, at least in primary schools, for which
women are especially fitted."[68] He notes Marshall's occupations for gentlemen
and points out that teachers come from "modest social class origin" compared
with the "elite professions."[69] He maintains that the work of teachers is based
on low expertise, does not create knowledge, has a holistic orientation to students, serves a compulsory population, uses simple language, has performance
that is hard to evaluate, and that it is performed in isolation. These are attributes that he also applies to nursing to justify his assertion of nursing (and
teaching) is an occupation rather than a profession. He writes that nurses

> transmit rather than create knowledge and perform their operations
> on captive, often intractable clients. Their language to patients has
> frequently to be simplified. …They are not as concerned as are
> teachers with the whole person. Their knowledge base is weak…
> the autonomy of the nurse, who is continually overseen at work and
> who can be seen at times by patients to be of lowly status, is far less
> than that of the teacher.[70]

Even granting that this is written in 1970, it seems to have had little actual
contact with nursing or knowledge of nursing history, and it appears to be
based in social and cultural stereotypes both of women and of nursing. Is there
hope that nursing might take its rightful place among the elite professions?

Tronto has at least a modicum of hope, not specifically that nursing will be viewed universally as a profession, but for a more basic social, specifically political, change—the expanding of moral boundaries to incorporate the terrain of caring. She believes that there is a way that caring can be incorporated into the political vision of the United States. Her claim is that "the practice of care describes the qualities necessary for democratic citizens to live together well in a pluralistic society, and that only in a just, pluralistic, democratic society can care flourish."[71] If care and care practices are accorded a core position in the democratic vision of the United States, it is likely that nursing too will be acknowledged as a core profession in contributing to that vision for the United States.

A Global Perspective on Nursing and the Societal View Approach

While the discussion has focused on nursing in the United States, the intersections of globalization, health, health care, gender, race, and class are mirrored globally. In a collaborative effort, *The Lancet*, the Harvard School of Public Health, and several other groups formed the Special Commission on Women and Health. Its charge: to reexamine existing evidence and to develop a strategic framework for a global agenda for women and health. The Women and Health Initiative (W&HI) was launched in 2010 to examine women's health needs and their paid and unpaid contributions to health care. More specifically, the W&HI focuses on two broad areas:

- Women's health throughout the life cycle, with an emphasis on the most neglected and urgent issues, such as maternal mortality, unsafe abortion, adolescents' sexual and reproductive health, contraception, gender-based violence and chronic diseases.

- Women in the healthcare system of which they are critical, yet under-recognized, pillars. W&HI studies the roles, responsibilities, and status of women at all levels of health systems: in the household, the community, the workforce, in academia, and as both formal and informal decision-makers and providers of care.[72]

The report of their study was released June 5, 2015. A summary of its findings are that

persistent social and gender inequality, violations of human rights (including the right to health care), and cultural backgrounds that perpetuate social injustice and limit women's human development, girls and women are at increased risk of ill health and have a low status in the health system, in which they have dual roles as both consumers and providers of health care.[73]

Additionally, the study states:

> Health systems are often unresponsive to the needs of women despite the fact that such systems rely heavily on women's contributions to health care, whether paid or unpaid. Worldwide, most health-care providers are women. ... However, female health-care providers are not working to their full potential because they are undervalued and under-supported by the systems in which they work. In the health-care system, women tend to have lower-skilled, lower-paid jobs than men.[74]

The staggering degree of women's contribution, paid and unpaid, to health care is of particular note. The Commission differentiated between paid and unpaid contributions and assigned a value to unpaid women's health care. Their conclusion:

> Women's contributions in the health-care labour force and their crucial roles in the health care of families and communities are drivers of the wealth and health of nations, but are still underappreciated; on the basis of an analysis of 32 countries accounting for 52% of the world's population, we estimated that the financial value of women's contributions in the health system in 2010 was 2.35% of global gross [GDP] for unpaid work and 2.47% of GDP for paid work—the equivalent of US$3.052 trillion.[75]

The Commission adds that

> overall, women's paid and unpaid contributions to the health sector amount to 3.57% of global GDP with the lower bound, minimum wage scenario or the equivalent of US$2.26 trillion. [Using] the average wages reported in 2010, women's contributions sum to 4.81% of global GDP or the equivalent of $3.05 trillion. Accounting for gender wage differentials and social security benefits, the value of unpaid and paid work increases considerably to 7.04% of global GDP or the equivalent of $4.47 trillion.[76]

This detailed study casts a strong light on many of the concerns in intersectionality—and nursing—and makes a series of recommendations, in the following four categories:

Value Women

- Ensure women's universal access to health care that is responsive to gender and the life course; states should use the maximum available resources to ensure availability, accessibility, and quality of health services to address women's comprehensive needs.

- Recognize women's paid and unpaid contributions as healthcare providers.

- Develop, implement, and enforce gender-responsive policies to support women in their diverse roles and enable them to integrate their social, biological, and occupational contributions.

Compensate Women

- Estimate the value of women's paid and unpaid contributions to health care and recompense their invisible subsidy to health systems and societies.

- Ensure that men and women receive equal compensation for equal work in health and other sectors.

Count Women

- Ensure that women are accounted for in quantification of the health workforce.

- Guarantee that sex-disaggregated civil, vital, and health statistics and survey data are obtained through national systems.

- Mandate that research studies enroll women and publish findings disaggregated by sex.

Be Accountable to Women

- Develop and implement an accountability framework and indicators for women and health.

- Establish independent mechanisms at global and country levels to support, catalyse, and ensure accountability for global, regional, and national action for women and health.[77]

It is interesting to note the nature of their argument. As the title of the article would indicate, the report concludes that "sustainable development needs women's social, economic, and environmental contributions, which will increase when women are healthy, valued, enabled, and empowered to reach their full potential in all aspects of their lives, including in their roles as providers of health care."[78] This is largely an economic argument: women need to be healthy reach their full potential to contribute to sustainable growth. While human rights are mentioned, and specifically the human rights of women, the report's fundamental argument is one of sustainable development.[79] Note its mention of human rights:

> Recognition, valuation, and compensation of women's roles in health care are necessary to achieve gender equality and maximise women's contributions to families, communities, and society. Not only will women be able to provide improved health care with increased support, but they will also be able to pursue education and production opportunities, thus advancing their fundamental human rights and contributing to sustainable development.[80]

In its Millennium Development Goals, the United Nations argues primarily from a human rights perspective but also include arguments rooted in dignity, peace, prosperity, and justice as well as sustainability.[81]

This study is significant in the context of nursing and the societal view approach: Nursing is the largest healthcare profession and, globally, it is female-dominant. At the global level, female healthcare labor remains undervalued, under-supported, utilized below its potential and preparation, and constrained by intersections of culture, power, and gender as well as race and class. We move now from the several approaches to defining professions to Johnson's perspective that defining professions is a misdirected effort.

Profession as One Type of Occupational Control

Terence Johnson, in *Professions and Power*, sees the entire enterprise of defining profession as ill-founded and misdirected. He maintains that "a profession is not an occupation, but a means of controlling an occupation."[82] His emphasis is on the nature of the relationship between the client/consumer and the professional/producer of labor. He argues for three fundamental relationships, specifically that there are three forms of occupational control: *collegiate, patronage,* and *mediative.* Aspects of all three forms of occupational control are evident in nursing. Collegiate control is that form that is associated with medicine, law, and clergy—that is, those groups that have classically been regarded as professions. In collegiate occupational control, the profession is self-policing; the profession determines its standards of education and practice; the professional determines when the professional relationship will begin and end, what transpires in the relationship, what the needs are and how they will be met. There is a great distance between the consumer and producer and the consumer has a high level of uncertainty regarding the content of the producer's discipline and no ability to judge the quality of the work. In addition, the consumer is dependent upon the producer. Dentistry would be a good example here. This form of occupational control is associated with those occupations generally socially regarded as professions.[83]

The patronage form of occupational control differs from the collegiate form in that it is the patron who determines when the relationship will start or stop, what the content or task of production is, and how that task will be accomplished. Social distance benefits the individual or corporate patron and uncertainty is reduced in favor of the patron/consumer. Johnson sees engineering and accounting as governed by patronage occupational control, but this category would also include architecture and art or craft.[84]

Mediative occupational control exists where a third party sets the terms of the relationship. It is the mediative control that determines when a relationship will begin or end, what needs will or will not be met, and how they will be met, who may be the producer, who may be the consumer, and what the choices are. It is Johnson's understanding that professions as they have been known, and as they have previously operated under collegiate control, are moving toward mediative occupational control. In essence, mediative occupational control restrains the autonomy of the producer, thus the traditional professions that understood autonomy as a chief defining characteristic are gradually losing significant degrees of autonomy. The intrusion of third-party payers in medicine and the state in a range of occupations is an example of growing mediative control. The corporatization of education and academic research would also fit this category (discussed in Chapter 4).[85] Nursing had and continues to have all three forms of occupational control operative in the sphere of nursing practice, though nursing education and research continue to operate more from a collegiate form of occupational control.

Of the various methods of assessing an occupation for its status as a profession, nursing meets the methodological standards for the first three approaches. The last three methods are sufficiently rooted in cultural and social bias that it

---

THINKING ABOUT OCCUPATIONAL CONTROL...

Of Johnson's three forms of occupational control (collegiate, patronage, and mediative), the collegiate form is associated with the classical professions, that is, those occupations socially and widely regarded as professions. The classical professions of law, medicine, and clergy—and maybe teaching—demonstrated considerable autonomy of practice, set their own standards for practice and education, and policed their own members. Collegiate occupational control, however, is eroding and professions are coming increasingly under mediative control. Today there are all sorts of mediative controllers that limit the health professional's autonomy: insurance systems, government programs, group practices, HMOs, PPOs, DRGs, and more. Might it be possible that one day mediative control will overtake all professions and they will cease to exist as we have known them?

is unlikely that nursing, teaching, and any female- or minority-dominant occupation would be deemed a profession, at least until there is significant social change. But defining professions is only one aspect that requires attention. The question of the role of professions in society still remains.

Two Approaches to the Role of Professions in Society
A Positive View

There are two general approaches to the role of professions in society. Durkheim maintains that as post-industrial society grew and evolved, pluralism grew; social ties were loosened and morality became less binding. For Durkheim, professions, by which he means all occupations, became the custodians of morality.[86] Professions, as they arose, provided an altruistic, self-policing, moral community that contributed to the integration of society and social order.[87] Larsen's interpretation is that "Durkheim could see in the organization of the professions not only the modern expression of the medieval corporations but also the social model that would produce the ethics and rules needed by a complex division of labor, and thus save modern society from the chronic anomie rooted in its economy."[88] *Anomie*, the social instability created by the lack of governing social or ethical standards, could be overcome as the professions created a new form of community and solidarity. This is a positive view of the role of professions in society and yet there are egregious examples of professions' power-brokering, failure at self-policing, failure of altruism, and exercise of pecuniary self-interest.[89]

A Cynical View

The second general approach to the role of professions in society is substantially more cynical and distrustful. This view, however, incorporates the abundance of evidence of professions' failures. In this view, professions are monopolistic power elites that use their specialized knowledge to wield and increase their social, political, and economic power through the exploitation of a grave social need. In this view, professions suppress competition, further their dominance and privilege, circumscribe their numbers, and fail at self-policing.[90]

The evidence would indicate that professions exist somewhere between these two extremes, though as we shall see in the next chapter, society has lost a degree of trust in a number of professions and views them as having broken faith with the public and in breach of their social contract. We shall come to that shortly, but to finish this discussion, the important question here is not so much how nursing lives out its role in society, but rather, "if nursing were an elite profession of great social, political, and economic power, how *might* it live out its role in society?" Based on nursing's history of balancing self-interest with service to society and patients, there is reason to believe that nursing would, under those conditions, attempt to move care to the center of political and social values. Here the reader is reminded of the exceptionally high level of social trust that society has for nursing, above that of other professions. That trust, in part, recognizes nursing's genuine commitment to care and to society.[91]

Nursing as a Profession

The nursing literature's self-reference is to nursing as a profession and NSPS takes nursing's status as a profession as a given. It notes that "nursing, like other professions, is an essential part of the society out of which it grew and within which it continues to evolve. Nursing is responsible to society in the sense that nursing's professional interest must be perceived as serving the interests of society."[92] In discussing the authority for nursing practice for nurses, NSPS declares that

> the authority for nursing, as for other professions, is based on social responsibility, which in turn derives from a complex social base and a social contract. …Nursing's social contract reflects the profession's long-standing core values and ethics, which provide grounding for health care in society. It is easy to overlook this social contract underlying the nursing profession when faced with certain facets of contemporary society, including depersonalization, apathy, discon-nectedness, and growing globalization. But upon closer examination,

---

THINKING ABOUT NURSING PROGRESS IN MY LIFETIME…

It is easy to get caught up in the woes of the current day when we think about the social status, power, and authority of nursing in 2015. Like watching your child grow, you don't see it until she or he needs new shoes or the jeans become high-water pants. It is the same with nursing—we don't see it grow until we realize we need a new specialty, perhaps zero-gravity or biosphere or interplanetary nursing. Talk to nurses of 40 or 50 years experience, nearing retirement. They may have grown up reading some or all of the 27 Cherry Ames mystery novels: Cherry Ames, Army Nurse; Cherry Ames, Chief Nurse; …Flight Nurse …Private Duty Nurse …Visiting Nurse …Night Supervisor Nurse …Mountaineer Nurse …Dude Ranch Nurse …Department Store Nurse, and more. When they entered nursing, intensive care units were experimental, there was no clinical specialization in nursing, nursing research was underfunded or had no funding at all, physicians still taught a number of nursing school courses, and nurses still wore caps, white (or blue) uniforms and white (or black) hose. Graduates in the 1960s could not have foreseen Master's-prepared clinical nurse specialists, congregational nurses, family nurse practitioners, transplant nurses, nurse legislators, or the National Institute of Nursing Research. They have witnessed profound changes in nursing as a profession.

To see nursing grow, write your own story, starting with the day of your graduation and continuing it to the day you retire. It will give you a long view of nursing's continuing development and great hope for its future as a profession. (The Cherry Ames nurse-mystery novels are still available in reprint from Springer Publishing Company: http://www.springerpub.com/nursing/cherry-ames-series.html.)

---

we see that society validates the existence of the profession through licensure, public affirmation, and legal and legislative parameters. Nursing's response is to provide care to all who are in need, regardless of their cultural, social, or economic standing.[93]

While some of the early modern nursing literature characterizes nursing as "becoming" a profession, the bulk of the literature does not—it already regards nursing as a profession. The public understanding of nursing, however, as well as medicine's understanding of nursing persisted in seeing it as an occupation even after nursing regarded itself as a profession. In addition, some of the sociological literature called nursing a semi-profession. These skirmishes have ceased and nursing has taken its place in society fully as a profession. However, as a profession that is care-based, it has fought and continues to fight for full recognition as a profession in all aspects. The battle looms large, as it entails changing the social location of women and minorities in the United States, the envaluing and centering of caring in the sociopolitical arena, and reforming within the profession regarding such issues as the entry points into practice. It is a daunting agenda, but no more difficult than what has been accomplished thus far from the beginning of nursing education in the early 1870s to the present.

ENDNOTES

All URLs provided are accurate as of May 29, 2015.

1   "Our History," St. Bartholomew's Hospital, http://www.bartshealth.nhs.uk/our-hospitals/st-bartholomew's-hospital/our-history/.

2   Alexander M. Carr-Saunders and Paul A. Wilson, *The Professions* (Oxford, UK: Oxford/Clarendon Press, 1933), 118.

3   Ibid., 117.

4   Ibid., 121.

5   "Nurse," The Internet Surname Database, http://www.surnamedb.com/Surname/Nurse.

6   Magali Safatti Larson, *The Rise of Professionalism: A Sociological Analysis* (Berkeley, CA: University of California, Berkeley Press, 1979), 15.

7   Adriano Tilgher, *Homo Faber: Work through the Ages*, (Washington, DC: Regnery/Gateway Editions, 1958). See also: Tilgher, *Work: What It Has Been to Men through the Ages*, trans. Dorothy C. Fisher (London: G. G. Harrap, 1931).

8   Marsha Fowler, "Is Occupational Labor a Spiritual Endeavor?" *The Park Ridge Center Bulletin* Winter 2001: 5–6.

9   John Calvin, *Institutes of the Christian Religion*, trans. Ford Lewis Battles (Philadelphia: Westminster Press, 1960), Book 3: *The Way in Which We Receive the Grace of Christ: What Benefits Come to Us from It, and What Effects Follow*, chapter 10, question 6, 1:724–25.

10   *Florence Nightingale to Her Nurses: A Selection from Miss Nightingale's Addresses to Probationers and Nurses of the Nightingale School at St. Thomas's Hospital* (London: Macmillan, 1914), 116.

11   Marsha Fowler, "Religion and Nursing," in *Religion, Religious Ethics and Nursing*, ed. Marsha Fowler et al. (New York: Springer, 2011), 13.

12   Lynn McDonald, ed., *Collected Works of Florence Nightingale*, vol. 3, *Florence Nightingale's Theology: Essays, Letters and Journal Notes* (Ontario: Wilfrid Laurier University Press, 2002), 74. See also: Gérard Vallée, ed., *Collected Works of Florence Nightingale*, vol. 4, *Florence Nightingale on Mysticism and Eastern Religions* (Ontario: Wilfrid Laurier University Press, 2006).

13   MacDonald, *Florence Nightingale's Theology*, 74–75.

14   Lynn McDonald, ed., *Collected Works of Florence Nightingale*, vol. 13, *Florence Nightingale: Extending Nursing* (Ontario: Wilfrid Laurier University Press, 2009), 752.

15   Hastings Rashdall, *The Universities of Europe in the Middle Ages*, ed. F. M. Powicke, and A. B. Emden, 3 vols., new ed. (Oxford: Clarendon Press, 1987).

16   Richard Hurd, ed., *The Works of the Right Honorable Joseph Addison in 6 Volumes*, vol. 2., new ed. (Covent Garden, England: Henry G. Bohn, 1856), 271.

17   Hilde de Ridder-Symoens,"Mobility," in *A History of the University in Europe*, ed. Walter Rüegg, vol. 1, *Universities in the Middle Ages* (Cambridge, UK: Cambridge University Press, 1992), 280–306. See also: Carr-Saunders and Wilson, *Professions*.

18   Graham Cheetham and Geoff Chivers, *Professions, Competence and Informal Learning* (Cheltenham, UK: Edward Elgar Publishing, 2005), 1.

19   John A. Jackson, ed., *Professions and Professionalization*, Sociological Studies 3 (Cambridge, UK: Cambridge University Press, 1970), 23.

20   Carr-Saunders and Wilson, *Professions*.

21   Eliot Freidson, *Professionalism: The Third Logic*, (Chicago: University of Chicago Press, 2001).

22   Geoffrey Millerson, "Education in the Professions," in *Education and the Professions*, ed. T.G. Cook (New York: Routledge, 1973), 1–18.

23   Cheetham and Chivers, *Professions, Competence and Informal Learning*, 4–10.

24   Margretta Styles, *On Nursing: Toward a New Endowment* (St. Louis, MO: CV Mosby, 1982). See also: Genevieve K. Bixler and Roy W. Bixler, "The Professional Status of Nursing," *American Journal of Nursing* 45, no. 9 (1945): 730–35; their reprise article: Bixler and Bixler, "The Professional Status of Nursing," *American Journal of Nursing* 59, no. 8 (1959): 1142–46; and M. N. Sleicher, "Nursing Is Not a Profession," *Nursing and Health Care* 2, no. 4 (April 1981): 186–92.

25 Abraham Flexner, *Medical Education in the United States and Canada: A Report to the Carnegie foundation for the Advancement of Teaching* (Boston: Marymount Press, 1910). See also: Carr-Saunders and Wilson, *Professions*; Bixler and Bixler, "Professional Status of Nursing" (1945); and Bixler and Bixler, "Professional Status of Nursing" (1959).

26 Marsha Fowler, "Social Ethics and Nursing," in *The Nursing Profession: Turning Points*, ed. Norma Chaska (St. Louis, MO: CV Mosby Company, 1990), 24–31.

27 Cheetham and Chivers, *Professions, Competence and Informal Learning*, 2–3.

28 Freidson, *Professionalism*, 90.

29 Ibid., 12.

30 Fowler, "Social Ethics and Nursing," 24. See also: Terence Johnson, *Professions and Power* (London, UK: Macmillan, 1972), 35–38.

31 Theodore Caplow, *The Sociology of Work*, (Minneapolis: University of Minnesota Press, 1954).

32 Howard Vollmer and Donald Mills, '*Professionalization*' (Englewood Cliffs, NJ: Prentice-Hall, 1966).

33 Harold Wilensky, "The Professionalization of Everyone?" *American Journal of Sociology* 70, no. 2 (September 1964): 137–48.

34 Ibid., 144–45.

35 Ibid., 142.

36 Ibid., 155.

37 T. H. Marshall, "The Recent History of Professionalism in Relation to Social Structure and Social Policy," *The Canadian Journal of Economics and Political Science* 5, no. 3 (August 1939): 325–40.

38 Ernest Greenwood, "Attributes of a Profession," *Social Work* 2, no. 3 (July 1957): 45–55.

39 Ibid.

40 Ibid., 46.

41 Ibid.

42 Talcott Parsons, "The Professions and Social Structure," *Social Forces* 17, no. 4 (May 1939): 457–67.

43 Greenwood, "Attributes of a Profession," 49.

44 Ibid., 50.

45 Ibid., 52.

46 Ibid., 53.

47 "Standard Occupational Classification," U.S. Government, http://www.bls.gov/soc/.

48 *Handbook of Occupational Groups and Families* (n.p.: U.S. Office of Personnel Management, 2009), http://www.opm.gov/policy-data-oversight/classification-qualifications/classifying-general-schedule-positions/occupationalhandbook.pdf.

49 "Introduction to occupational classifications," International Standard Classification of Occupations (ISCO), http://www.ilo.org/public/english/bureau/stat/isco/intro.htm.

50 *Statutory Instruments: The European Communities Professional Qualifications (Recognition of Professional Qualifications) Regulations 2007* (UK: The Stationery Office Limited, 2007), http://www.gmc-uk.org/European_Communities__Recognition_of_Professional_Quals__Regs.pdf_25392267.pdf.

51 "29-1141 Registered Nurses," Standard Occupational Classification, last updated March 11, 2010, http://www.bls.gov/soc/2010/soc291141.htm.

52 "ISCO-88: Major Group 3 Technicians and Associate Professionals; 31.323 Nursing and Midwifery Associate Professionals," LABORSTA Internet, http://laborsta.ilo.org/applv8/data/isco88e.html; See also: "ISIC Rev.4 code 8690," United Nations Statistics Division, http://unstats.un.org/unsd/cr/registry/regcs.asp?Cl=27&Lg=1&Co=8690.

53 Cheetham and Chivers, *Professions, Competence and Informal Learning*, 9.

54 Eliot Freidson, *Professional Power: A Study of the Institutionalization of Formal Knowledge* (Chicago: University of Chicago Press, 1986), 58.

55 Ibid., 9–10.

56 "Compare different qualifications," gov.UK, https://www.gov.uk/what-different-qualification-levels-mean/compare-different-qualification-levels.

57 Anthony Russell, *The Clerical Profession* (London: SPCK, 1980).

58 Ibid.

59 Cheetham and Chivers, *Professions, Competence and Informal Learning*, 10–11.

60 Barbara Melosh, *The Physician's Hand*, (Philadelphia: Temple University Press, 1982), 19.

61 Ibid., 20.

62 Fred Davis, ed., *The Nursing Profession: Five Sociological Essays* (New York: Wiley and Sons, 1966), 8.

63 "Fact Sheet: Enhancing Diversity in the Nursing Workforce," American Association of Colleges of Nursing, updated January 21, 2014, http://www.aacn.nche.edu/media-relations/diversityFS.pdf.

64 Ibid.

65 Author's note: Eileen Boris and Rhacel Parrenas, *Intimate Labors: Cultures, Technologies, and the Politics of Care* (Palo Alto, CA: Stanford University Press, 2010).

66 Marsha D. M. Fowler, *Guide to the Code of Ethics for Nurses: Development, Interpretation, and Application*, 2nd ed. (Silver Spring, MD: American Nurses Association, 2015), 31.

67 T. Leggatt, "Teaching as a Profession," in Jackson, *Professions and Professionalization*, 163–64.

68 Ibid., 164–65.

69 Ibid. See also: Marshall, "The Recent History of Professionalism," 325–40.

70 Leggatt, "Teaching as a Profession," 175–76.

71 Tronto, *Moral Boundaries*, 157–80.

[72] "Women and Health Initiative: Home," Harvard School of Public Health Women and Health Initiative, http://www.hsph.harvard.edu/women-and-health-initiative/.

[73] Ana Langer et al., "Women and Health: The Key for Sustainable Development," *Lancet*, published online June 5, 2015, 4, http://dx.doi.org/10.1016/S0140-6736(15)60497-4.

[74] Ibid., 2.

[75] Ibid., 1.

[76] Ibid., 27.

[77] Ibid., 2.

[78] Ibid., 1.

[79] Ibid., 1, 21, 30, 34.

[80] Ibid., 28, 30.

[81] Ban Ki-Moon, "Report of the UN Secretary-General: A Life of Dignity for All," un.org, http://www.un.org/millenniumgoals/pdf/SG_Report_MDG_EN.pdf.

[82] Johnson, *Professions and Power*, 57.

[83] Ibid.

[84] Ibid.

[85] Ibid.

[86] Theodore Steeman, "Durkheim's Professional Ethics," *Journal for the Scientific Study of Religion* 2, no. 2 (1963): 163–81.

[87] Émile Durkheim, *The Division of Labor in Society*, trans. Lewis Coser (New York: Free Press/Simon and Schuster, 1997). See also: Durkheim, *Professional Ethics and Civic Morals*, trans. Cornelia Brookfield (London: Routledge, 1957).

[88] Magali Sarfatti Larsen, *The Rise of Professionalism: A Sociological Analysis* (Berkeley: University of California Press, 1977), 54.

[89] See, for example: Henry K. Beecher, "Ethics and Clinical Research," *New England Journal of Medicine* 274, no. 24 (June 16, 1966): 1354–60; Allan J. McDonald and James Hansen, *Truth, Lies, and O-Rings: Inside the Space Shuttle Challenger Disaster* (Gainesville: University of Florida Press, 2009); and William O. Lowrance, *Of Acceptable Risk: Science and the Determination of Safety* (Los Altos, CA: William Kaufmann, 1976).

[90] Fowler, "Social Ethics and Nursing," 25.

[91] "Public Ranks Nurses," NursingWorld.org.

[92] ANA, *Nursing's Social Policy Statement*, 3.

[93] Ibid., 5.

Chapter 3.
Broken Professions
and How to Mend Them

Professions are out of place in today's society. They are a throwback to the industrial–manufacturing days of the United States. Professions have functioned largely autonomously within a social expectation of keeping faith with the public and the production of the social good for which they were specifically authorized by their social contract. Yet, society has found professions in breach of that social contract and out of faith with the public. This is in part a consequence of the changes in the social context of professions, and of the vicissitudes of the emergence of what has been called the new economy. Professions need repair through a course correction. By reclaiming their tradition of civic professionalism, professions will once again move public service, the welfare of the public, and the professional–public partnership, to the heart of their involvement with society. For medicine and nursing, doing so will further the realization of social goods such as health, solidarity, equality, equity, and dignity.

Professions and the New Economy

In today's society, professions are anachronistic. They are inconsistent with developing patterns of occupational labor that flex, morph, and transmute in the alchemy of the marketplace economy that has emerged over the past 30 years. But to understand why professions are odd in today's context, it is important to understand something about the new economy.

Historically there have been three economic sectors, each referring to a different category of economic activity (or "process of production"). In the U.S. Census Bureau's North American Industry Classification System (NAICS), the three major sectors are:[1]

Primary: Associated with agriculture, forestry, fishing, hunting, mining (277 subsectors)[2]

Secondary: Associated with manufacturing, including food, grain, textiles, clothing, wood, paper, printing, petroleum and its products, chemicals, rubber, pesticides, soap, plastic, clay, glass, concrete, iron, steel, machinery, and more (652 subsectors)[3]

Tertiary: Associated with service; also called the service sector (1280 subsectors)

The Service Sector

The attribute of the service sector is that it offers a range of services, that is, *activities*, not *products*. The service sector includes banking, entertainment, health care, information technology, professional services such as counseling or accounting, spectator sports, mass media, architecture, and more. Each of these produces a service, an intangible good, for a company (corporation) or for an individual. Health care and nursing are part of the service sector and, in the NAICS, Health Care and Social Assistance section of classification, are sector 62, with 92 subsectors. The healthcare sector includes a cluster of healthcare-related sectors: health system, healthcare industry, healthcare research, healthcare financing, healthcare administration, and regulation and health information technology. What is important to note here is the comparative number of subsectors in each category. Service sector occupations now greatly outnumber those of the manufacturing sector by almost 2:1.

The industrial–manufacturing (secondary) sector has waned and the service sector has grown. The NAICS Economic Classification Policy Committee notes several reasons for this:

> Service industries have become much more important than they were. …Services have not just grown in importance; radical changes have taken place in the nature of services produced in the economy. Some of the changes affecting services include the following:

- Technological changes, particularly in terms of computers, information, and communication services;

- Changes in intangible inputs, such as education, training and the growth of knowledge, which have increasingly become the basis for services transactions;

- Changes in government policy, such as decreased regulation of transportation and financial services;

- Contracting out of services (especially manufacturing);

- Changes in demographics, such as aging, and the consequent demand for health care, and;

- Changing consumption patterns and living standards, more consumption of entertainment, recreational and travel services, and so forth.[4]

Many of the changes that have given rise to the service sector over manufacturing are evident in our own lives as, for example, we have moved from corded to cordless phones, then to mobile phones, then to mobile phones connected to desktop computers, then connected to tablet computers, from which we can now watch television programs, movies, read books, or access library resources. Remembering, not imagining, is all that we need to see how we ourselves have witnessed the rise of the service and technology sector. Nurses who graduated in the 1960s and are now transitioning into retirement remember when intensive care units (ICUs) did not exist except as experimental units. They will remember when ICUs (primitive by today's standards) moved into non-teaching hospitals. In those days, one might see medical and surgical patients, adult and pediatric patients, and gynecologic and cardiac patients all in the same "intensive care unit." Soon thereafter nursing specializations would explode. Today, the ANA has standards of practice and professional performance for 22 nursing specialties; it will not stop there![5] *Nursing's Social Policy Statement* notes that

> the Standards of Professional Performance describe a competent level of behavior in the professional role, including activities related to quality of practice, education, professional practice evaluation, collegiality, collaboration, ethics, research, resource utilization, and leadership. Registered nurses are accountable [in all roles and venues] for their professional actions to themselves, their patients, their peers, and ultimately to society.[6]

That society has changed profoundly. It has moved from an agrarian to a manufacturing to a service society, and from a largely rural to a largely urban population. The Industrial Revolution moved the United States from hand-made production to manufacturing. In the United States, the Industrial Revolution begins in the founding of the Slater textile mill in the 1790s. Textiles moved from home and crafts production to industrial production. The United States moved from horse power (real horses!) to water power to steam power and eventually to coal power. The first phase of the Industrial Revolution continued to about 1850. It got a second wind in 1855 with the patenting of the Bessemer process for steel production. Though the dates are contested, the Industrial Revolution ends with World War I. We are now a post-industrial society in which the economy has, in great measure, shifted from a manufacturing to a service economy. Modern nursing emerged during the Civil War, during the end of the first portion of the Industrial Revolution and the beginning of the second. The reader is encouraged to look at the fascinating period of nursing history between the Civil War and World War I when nursing moves both into private duty nursing in the home, and into society as advocates for public health. Today's social context of nursing is not that of our forbearers: it is a service and technological economy and society in which nursing has grown into increasingly complex and advanced roles.

The New Economy

The new economy refers to the shift that has taken place in the economy as the United States has transitioned from an industrial/manufacturing economy to one based on service and information technology. The manufacturing economy brought with it job security, a life-long employer, regular wages, a rising income scale, health benefits, pension systems, career ladders, job stability, and more. The new economy, on the other hand, is much more volatile and much less secure occupationally. It is characterized by entrepreneurship, rapid change, distributed management, continuous innovation, skill flexibility, teamwork, continuous learning, risk, networking, contingency, and more. Williams and colleagues describe this environment: "In the so-called new economy, work is increasingly characterized by job insecurity, teamwork, career maps and networking."[7]

Professions do not have a good fit with the new economy and the new workplace. Sullivan writes that

> the traditional structures of professional life, such as corporate membership [professional associations], controlled markets for professional services, and monopolistic practices in training, recruitment and the control of standards, seem quaint and even antithetical to some of the most touted new patterns of work. The question is: "Where do the professions fit in the future depicted as a globalizing march toward a *frictionless capitalism* that is based upon information and communications technology?" The fluid morphing of one occupational identity for another and the migration of disparate domains of activity celebrated as a *new economy* are antithetical at a number of points with key elements of professionalism. Today's enthusiasm for untrammeled flexibility in workers is not a good match with the professions' demand for deep training in a complex under-determined field that requires professional judgment and integrity. Professions, unlike businesses, are pledged to protect those in vulnerable situations.[8]

Issues emerge here that are not our immediate concern but need to be mentioned, such as the demand for nurses to work (float) disparate domains of clinical activity, or the pressure for more rapid production or graduation of nurses, and the pressure to reduce educational requirements for nursing in the direction of manualism. The present concern, however, is for the place and future of professions in the context of radical socioeconomic change. Despite their anachronistic status, professions persist in society, even in the new economy, though, as Sullivan notes, professions are broken and in need of repair.

Professions: Breaking Faith with the Public and in Breach of Contract

In addition to being an anachronism, Sullivan reproaches the professions for their part in breakdowns of "core sectors in the emerging new economy," much of the "breakdown of public oversight," and destructive deregulation. He cites the "US financial bubble burst" and the Enron scandal that directly implicates professionals in law, accounting, and banking. He writes that, "quite correctly, both officials and the public saw the leading lawyers and accountants of those organizations as guilty of an insolent repudiation of public trust."[9] He notes a public "suspicion that professionals have broken faith with the public" more generally.[10]

Breaking Faith

The Enron and banking crises are not the only examples of professions breaking faith with the public and breaching the social contract. There are examples across many professions, many of which have claimed mass media attention.

THINKING ABOUT THE START OF THE NEW ECONOMY...

In her book *Animal, Vegetable, Miracle: A Year of Food Life*, Barbara Kingsolver writes of her experience of taking her family into dietary near self-sufficiency. For a year her family ate only what they could grow themselves on a farm in Southern Appalachia or could obtain locally. They learned sowing and growing and harvesting plants and animals, canning foods, the vicissitudes of raising turkeys, how to make cheese, and on and on. They ate only what was in season, and swapped with local residents for things they did not grow. So: no strawberries in January and no avocados at all. Only if they had canned it could they eat it out of season. They became locavores. Except for flour and cooking oil, which they could neither produce themselves nor obtain locally.

That was the glitch in their self-sufficiency. Even for those of us who have dabbled in hobbies of soap making, candle making, furniture making, spinning, weaving, sewing, leather tanning, basket making, foraging, cooking over fire, and who had neighbors who engaged in other useful hobbies, we still do not achieve self-sufficiency. But that's okay. It can be ordered. On the Internet. From Germany. As economies have become increasingly intertwined and interdependent, so have individuals, families, communities, nations, none of which are self-sufficient. Neither are professions.

Both Beecher and Pappworth have noted ethical violations in medical research in the United States and the United Kingdom, respectively.[11]

In 1966, Henry Beecher's landmark paper on ethics in human research was published.[12] Beecher, an anesthesiologist, identifies 22 medical research projects that were conducted by prestigious universities, published in respected medical journals, and were deeply ethically questionable. The paper makes for very disturbing, even frightening, reading. In addition to the 22 experiments that Beecher identifies in the paper (and many others that were not in the paper), there were a number of studies that became well-known and roused public ire. Four such studies included the Willowbrook experiment, the Tuskegee experiment, the Tearoom Trade experiment, and the Milgram obedience experiment.[13]

Two additional examples are the Ford Pinto gas tank explosions, and the Challenger Shuttle O-ring failure. In the case of the Ford Pinto car there was a design flaw in the placement of the gas tank as well as economizing measures in its construction and mount that proved dangerous. In rear collisions over 25 miles per hour, a bolt would puncture the gas tank and cause fuel leakage that could spark, cause the gas tank to enflame and the passengers to suffer severe burn injuries or burn deaths. The flaw was discovered during testing, but in Ford's risk–benefit analysis the decision was made that it would cost more to re-tool and correct the flaw than to compensate victims for burn injuries or death.[14] It was criticized that in Ford's profit-based risk–benefit equation, human life was accorded insufficient value.

The second example took place in 1986 when the space shuttle *Challenger* disintegrated shortly after launch, killing all seven crew members aboard. An O-ring seal (made by Morton Thiakol) in the right rocket booster had failed, ultimately causing a structural failure that lead aerodynamic forces to break the shuttle apart. The launch, and subsequent disaster, had been widely covered by the media and was witnessed by millions of Americans on television. An investigating commission found that the flaws in the O-ring seals (which would fail under a certain ambient temperature level) were known, that the disaster could have been avoided, and that it was largely a consequence of NASA organizational culture and decision-making processes that ignored warnings and did not adequately communicate engineering–technical concerns.[15]

Reclaiming a Moral Force

Sullivan's analysis of the failures on the part of professionals is much broader than simple avarice and dereliction. Much like Durkheim, he characterizes professions as a moral force for good in society, a force that needs to be reclaimed. His starting point in that reclamation is the belief that professions offer something of moral value to society:

I argue that a democratic society also draws heavily on the skills and moral sources of the professions. Particularly within a society like ours, in which the pull of utility and instrumental thinking—as in today's ascendant *business model* for institutions—is so strong, the professions are vital reminders that human welfare ultimately depends upon cultivation of values such as care and responsibility, which cannot be produced by self-interest alone. By focusing on the quality of their craft and the inventiveness of their practice, professionals provide an alternative model of what work can be: a contribution to public value, as well as a source of motivation and deep personal satisfaction.[16]

The privileged position of professions in society is based on a social contract from which a number of expectations arise. Those include establishing standards of practice and education, ethical behavior, competence, a degree of altruism, responsibility and accountability, self-policing, and the like as discussed in earlier chapters. As NSPS notes, "the professions are expected to act responsibly, always mindful of the public trust."[17] Sullivan writes, "professionals are often engaged in generating or applying new ideas and advanced processes, and so are doing 'creative' work, that are all directly pledged to an ethic of public service."[18] According to Sullivan, professions are to engage in a partnership with society where the profession is accountable and responsible and the public is actively engaged and concerned: "These are the stakeholders of the various professional enterprises in health, justice, education and the rest. [This]…ideal of social reciprocity is called *civic professionalism*."[19] (The issue of stakeholders will become important for Chapter 4.) He cites Brint's work that points to "a long-term movement away from an earlier conception of professionalism as 'social trusteeship.' The drift is toward embracing a notion of the professional as a purveyor of expert services. …The term *technical professionalism* is employed to refer to this tendency."[20]

Sullivan's claim is that "the narrowing of professional claims toward the purely cognitive or technical in recent decades has contributed to the weakening of professionalism,"[21] resulting in a decline in professional civic engagement, a loss of concern for the welfare of society, a decline in altruism and professional ethics, and the reconceptualization of the recipient as consumer of a commodity. He calls for several changes to move professionals away from technical and into civic professionalism.

Restoring a Sense of Calling

One such change is the restoration of a sense of calling or vocation among professionals, to strengthen a professional culture of altruism and commitment to the public good.[22] Here, vocation as calling must be distinguished from *vocationalism*, a skills-based technicalism, with no roots in calling. In reclaiming the concept of vocation, the profession becomes a part of the person's identity, the work meaningful as "love of craft," and the occupation more than just a job. Sullivan's claim is that "it is 'affection for the subject matter,' the particular domain of professional activity that motivates and consolidates love of craft into 'a standing disposition' to serve."[23] This is the nurse who loves nursing and who finds satisfaction, if not joy, in service. Vocation is not only essential to civic professionalism, it also removes the possibility of runaway self-interest on the part of the professional.

There is more that is needed for professional reform. The outcome of the professional's work must "contribute to the public value for which the profession stands."[24] For its part, the public, in this profession–public partnership, must take leadership in resolving issues of abuse of privilege and the professions' refusal of public accountability.[25] He calls upon physicians not to recast "patients as consumers" or to "narrow professional roles to fit short-term encounters."[26] He goes further in this project of reform by tackling professional education, calling upon it to recover the formative dimension of professional culture, character, and values.[27] He identifies three sets of values: "Values of the academy, the values of professional practice, and the ethical-social values of professional identity."[28] Sullivan particularly emphasizes the last. He writes that

> this third set of values emphasizes the professional's integrity, sense of direction, and ability to assume responsibility for the quality of his or her own work and the standards associated with the field of practice. These values ground professional education in a broader conception of the purpose of the profession and the ideals to which it aspires, connecting training directly with the field's social contract.[29]

Sullivan's summative argument is that

> professionalism has proven an ambiguous good. The ambiguity stems in large measure from professionalism's loss of direction. This in turn has been due to weakening connections between the professions and the culture of civic democracy. …The professional life can and needs to be restructured in ways that suffuse technical competence with civic awareness and purpose.[30]

Citizenship in Nursing

Nursing has a long history of a call to civic awareness and participation and to fulfilling the duties of citizenship. While early discussions of the duties of citizenship presumed actual legal citizenship, they also understood citizenship as a larger construct referring to *civitas*, the body of all contributing members of the society, irrespective of legal status. For the purposes of this work, citizenship should be understood as the latter, and as having no reference to immigration status. It is beyond the compass of this chapter to present a detailed account of nursing's concern for civic participation, which can be found extensively in the nursing literature (both books and journal articles) from the late 1800s to the present. However, a few examples taken from the various revisions of the Code will give evidence of nursing's concern for participatory citizenship by nurses, specifically as nurse–citizens.

Citizenship and the Code of Ethics for Nurses

The *Suggested Code* of 1926 details five relational categories of moral duties of the nurse. They are: nurse to patient, nurse to the medical profession, nurse to allied professions, nurse to nurse, and nurse to her (exclusively) profession. However, the preamble of the *Suggested Code* sets all five of these relationships of moral obligation within the larger umbrella context of nursing's relationship to society. It states:

> Nursing emerges as a profession from its historic setting in an attempt to meet the present demands of society. The most precious possession of this profession is the ideal of service extending even to the sacrifice of life itself, in its incessant effort to meet the need of the world. …The nurse is primarily a citizen. The fundamental basis of ethics is the same for every profession. The obligation of each individual is to serve society as well as possible by contributing that for which he is best fitted. The obligation of society is to see that the individual has the opportunity to develop and to realize the fullest health and happiness possible without interfering with others.[31]

Without using the term *social contract*, the passage nonetheless contains social contract language, bringing together elements of the social contract in citizenship, society's need/the world's need, altruistic service, citizenship, ethics, reciprocal obligation, social contribution, and more.

The *Tentative Code* of 1940 contains a defense of nursing as a profession, detailing the attributes of a profession and how it is that nursing demonstrates them. This is not material that belongs in a proper code of ethics, but it does reflect the concern of nursing that it be externally counted among the professions. The sixth attribute of a profession ("a well-knit professional organization") contains this statement: "The professional spirit may be defined as a sense of responsibility for social advancement which will tend to inspire public respect and support for the profession."[32] This proposed code contains a substantive section on the nurse's relation to the public. It states, in part, because the nurse is a good citizen and because her professional preparation especially qualifies her…she will participate according to her ability, in those local and national activities that are carried on for social improvement. [The nurse will] …do her part in securing and enforcing laws, sustaining institutions, and promoting new measures which will advance the interests of humanity.[33]

Nursing is concerned for patients and for the health of society. But it is also concerned for the general welfare of society, indeed, for all of humanity, in ways not solely tied to health. The proposed codes of 1926 and 1940 were written in narrative form. The first code of ethics adopted by the ANA in 1950, the *Code for Professional Nurses* contains a preamble and an enumerated list of 17 provisions. The preamble states this: "Service to mankind is the primary function of nurses and the reason for the existence of the nursing profession. …Inherent in the code is the fundamental concept that the nurse subscribes to the democratic values to which our country is committed."[34] Three provisions are particularly important to the concept of citizenship and civic engagement—and democracy:

> *Provision 15.* The nurse as a citizen understands and upholds the laws and as a professional worker is especially concerned with those laws which affect the practice of medicine and nursing.

> *Provision 16.* A nurse should participate and share responsibility with other citizens and health professions in promoting efforts to meet the health needs of the public—local, state, national, and international.

> *Provision 17.* A nurse recognizes and performs the duties of citizenship, such as voting and holding office when eligible; these duties include an appreciation of the social, economic, and political factors which develop a desirable pattern of living together in a community.[35]

Re-Shaping Society

These themes continue in successive revisions of the Code. The rise of the field of bioethics in the late 1960s, with its emphasis on principles (respect for autonomy, nonmaleficence, beneficence, and justice), deeply affects the language and emphases of the Code from 1985 on. While concerns for the public remain, explicit references to nurses' duties of citizenship disappear. In 2001, however, citizenship and civic engagement make a comeback in Provision 9: "The profession of nursing, as represented by associations and their members, is responsible for articulating nursing values, for maintaining the integrity of the profession and its practice, and for shaping social policy."[36] The provision's interpretive statements incorporate the functions of social ethics (which will be discussed in Chapter 4). The focus of this provision is largely upon the role of the profession, through its associations, in shaping society, social and health policy, and social reform. To accomplish this, "nurses can work individually as citizens or collectively through political action to bring about social change."[37] While this and previous codes speak of the duties of citizenship, they are always placed within a context that conceives of this as nurse-as-citizen, not nurse-and-citizen. That is to say that all, both citizen and nurse, comingle to compose one's nursing identity. Remember that calling or vocation brings about a fusing of personal and professional identity and values; they become inseparable.

In part through its historic concern for public health, socially disadvantaged persons, and the social determinants of illness that have created health disparities, nursing has increased its ethical emphasis on civic engagement and civic professionalism since the 1985 Code. Again, the 2001 Code calls upon nursing organizations

> to speak collectively for nurses in shaping and reshaping health care within our nation, specifically in areas of healthcare policy and legislation. …In these activities health is understood as being broader than delivery and reimbursement systems, but extending to health-related sociocultural issues such as violation of human rights, homelessness, hunger, violence and the stigma of illness.[38]

Civic Engagement as an Intrinsically Political Act

Civic engagement refers to carrying the values and ideals of nursing into political action. While *technical professionalism* focuses on the acquisition, mastery, and implementation of the technical knowledge and skills of nursing in the delivery of patient care, *civic professionalism* sets nursing and nursing care within

---

THINKING ABOUT NURSING AS A CALLING…

It was not so very long ago that little girls were told that they could be a teacher, nurse, or secretary when they grew up. Today little girls can dream about being anything they want, and little boys can now dream about being a nurse. They may flit from wanting to be one thing to another, sometimes not even occupations. Little Kathy wanted to be an airplane when she grew up. Some of these children settle on nursing at an early age, and some later—its all that they want to be, and when they get there its all that they ever wanted to be. It is a sense of direction and determination that is inexplicable, it just *is*. As they mature, these persons have a sense of nursing as a calling. Nursing is a tough, high stakes job. It demands knowledge, skill, excellence, vigilance, creativity, resilience, physical energy, and more. The hours or schedule can be bad, the pay mediocre, the demands stiff, the patients irascible, and tragedies abound. For the nurse who has a sense of calling, even amidst all that is difficult, there is still a sense of satisfaction in the nature of what one is doing. Without that sense of calling, it is simply grinding, inexorable, frustration and toil.

---

the broader moral, social, and political context that is concerned to advance or reform health and health care. Boyte and Fretz write of the task of civic engagement as engendering "civic professionals who will renew a robust sense of the public purposes of their work and will develop and sustain a far more public culture for collaborative, visible, open work."[39] Nursing has never lost the "robust sense of public purpose of [its] work." However, the 2015 Code amplifies that role in several ways, calling nurses to engagement that serves the common good, seeks social justice, raises international health diplomacy to parity with economic and other concerns, leads collaborative efforts for health policy and legislation that positively impacts health, protects human rights, and addresses the structural, social, and institutional inequalities and disparities that are damaging to health and well-being.[40] While every nurse is called upon to contribute, no one nurse can meet these obligations alone. Civic engagement through civic professionalism requires collaborative and united efforts among nurses and with other health professions, activists, and organizations.[41]

Civic Professionalism and Nursing

Civic professionalism puts public service, the welfare of the public, and the professional–public partnership at the heart of the profession's involvement with society. It seeks to further social goods such as health, solidarity, equality, equity, and dignity. This raises two pivotal questions: "How does nursing further develop its civic professionalism?" and "How does nursing go about engaging in civic professionalism?"

Developing Civic Professionalism Through Education

Central to Sullivan's enterprise of restoring civic professionalism to professions is a renewal of university education for the professions with the analytic habits of mind that it cultivates.[42] What he advocates is combining that analytic formation with the best aspects of apprenticeship, "initiation into the wisdom of practice," through a "pedagogy of modeling expert judgement and then coaching the learner through similar activities," that works to form a "clinical habit of mind."[43] What he calls for is a blend of the analytic with the practical in a *cognitive apprenticeship*. This cognitive apprenticeship has three "large chunks" as he calls them: (a) intellectual or cognitive apprenticeship as found in the university context, (b) "imagined or simulated practice situations" taught by competent practitioners, and (c) an introduction of students to "the values and attitudes shared by the professional community" by teaching "the skills and traits, along with the ethical comportment, social roles, and responsibilities that mark the professional."[44]

Sullivan explicitly addresses nursing education, drawing heavily upon the work of Patricia Benner. He writes that

the essential goal of the professional school must be to form practitioners who are aware of what it takes to become competent in
their chosen domain and equip them with the reflective capacity and
motivation to pursue genuine expertise. In the case of nursing, for
example, this would mean studying and understanding the changing
conditions of practice, as illuminated by history and the social sciences, alongside the study of the field's particular knowledge base in
the physical sciences. ...Identification and formation of skillful ethical comportment must be the organizer of competence and inspira-
tion of expert work.[45]

He goes on to say that

the third apprenticeship ["chunk"] of professional identity has to pre-
cede and interpenetrate the learning of formal analytic knowledge in
the first apprenticeship and the development of skilled practice in
the second. To neglect formation in the meanings of the community,
and the larger public purposes for which the profession stands is to
risk educating mere technicians for hire in place of genuine
professionals.[46]

The Necessity of a Liberal Education

Roth, who advocates for liberal education as essential, points to the necessity of
incorporating liberal education in our modes of teaching in higher education.
In the midst of increasing cultural diversity of the nation and nursing's call for

---

THINKING ABOUT CIVIC PROFESSIONALISM...

Henry J. Kaiser, a renowned 20th-century industrialist, established shipyards that built, among
other craft, the Liberty ships, cargo vessels that his workers could build within five days, during
World War II. During that war, he also developed Kaiser Permanente Health Care to meet the
health needs of his shipyard workers and their families, and went on to found Kaiser Aluminum,
Kaiser Steel, and the Kaiser Foundation. After his first wife died, Henry married Beth, a nurse. In
1947, they established the Kaiser Foundation School of Nursing.

Beth's favorite color was pink. For decades, Kaiser cement trucks were locally renowned for
being painted a very, very hot pink. You could hear the wet cement grinding around as the giant
mixing barrels turned on the truck. The motto printed on the barrel read "Find a need and fill it."
The monstrous barrel slowly rotated and the motto would cycle 'round and 'round and 'round as
the trucks lumbered through the Bay Area. For a large construction project, there might be a slow
snaking conga line of pink trucks clogging the city grid. Perhaps it is stereotyping, but one would
expect these gargantuan trucks to be driven by big and burly types. Look closely, if only in your
mind. One is driven by Florence Nightingale. Another by Edith Cavell. One by Mary Mahoney. Is
that a Kaiser Permanente nurse driving the next? "Find a need and fill it": civic professionalism,
truckin' on down the road.

---

cultural humility, as well as nursing's recognition of the social determinants of health and the social disadvantaging of vulnerable populations, Roth's words are particularly important in relation to the "third apprenticeship":

> Contemporary liberal education should do more than supplement critical thinking with empathy and a desire to understand others from their own points of view. We should also supplement our strong critical engagement with social and cultural norms by developing modes of teaching that allow our students to enter in the value-laden practices of a particular culture to understand better how these values are legitimated: how the values are lived as legitimate. Current thinking in the humanities is often strong at showing that values that are said to be shared are really imposed on more vulnerable members of a particular group. Current thinking in the humanities is also good at showing the contextualization of norms, whether the context is generated by an anthropological, historical, or formal disciplinary matrix.[47]

Barriers: Corporatization of Education and Research

While Sullivan, and Benner and colleagues, correctly identify the need for education in civic professionalism, there are significant interrelated barriers to achieving this generally, and in nursing specifically. First, as Sullivan notes, there has been a corporatization of higher education, an issue to which he gives only passing attention. The effects of the corporatization of higher education upon nursing education, practice, and professionalism have yet to be explored. Corporatization of the university is "the adoption of business-related values and practices and the commercialization of faculty research."[48] Michael Crow, executive vice provost at Columbia University has claimed that universities "are expanding what it means to be a knowledge enterprise. We use knowledge as a form of venture capital."[49] For Bailey and Freedman,

> it is a picture of renewed privatisation, intensive marketisation, rampant financialisation and a challenge to the very notion of the university as a mechanism for addressing social inequality and facilitating the circulation of knowledge whether or not it has immediate practical consequences. It is the substitution of private economic activity for robust public life.[50]

Schrecker points out the 70% of college-level education is taught by "contingent faculty members" (adjunct faculty not holding a regular faculty appointment), the implications of which "for the quality of its instruction, for the welfare of its students, and for the university's ability to carry out its traditional mission—can only be disastrous."[51] Her observation is that more than money is at stake here. One can envision a dystopic set of institutions, dominated by vocationalism and the bottom line, where the drive for productivity transforms most faculty members into temporary workers with little job security or control over the content of their courses, while scientists and engineers churn out patentable results in industrialized laboratories that service their corporate sponsors. Such a constricted model of the academic community not only would stunt the careers and futures of students and teachers but also would undermine the very idea of the university as a place for intellectual growth and meaningful scholarship. Academic freedom is in danger here, as is the future of the well-informed citizenry that our democratic system requires. An academy transformed into a site for job training and corporate research will be increasingly hard-pressed to retain its function as the last remaining haven for reasoned dissent and the home of serious ideas that do not lend themselves to sound bites.[52]

The potential consequences that the corporatization of research has for nursing research are disturbing. Corporate research is geared toward the scientific generation of patentable, marketable results. When states and the federal government decrease research spending, relying instead on the corporate support of research, nursing research is largely endangered. Studies of quality of life, suffering, grief, coping, health disparities, and all the concerns of nursing tend not to produce patentable, marketable results.

In terms of the corporatization of education, what is at stake here is not simply the job security of professors, nor the integrity of academic research, though both are seen as being imperiled. Note that, in a larger vision, what is at stake is intellectual growth and meaningful scholarship, research devoted to the advance of a discipline, academic freedom—in short, those elements of education essential to an informed citizenry and to democracy itself. The threats to democracy itself are persistent themes in the literature of the emerging field of critical university studies. Few views of the corporatization of education are temperate from the academic side. Bailey and Freedman echo Schrecker in their assessment of the effects of laissez-faire economics on the university:

> More profoundly, it has weakened if not nearly destroyed those institutions that enable the production of a *formative culture* in which individuals learn to think critically, imagine other ways of being and doing, and connect their personal troubles with public concerns. Matters of justice, ethics and equality have once again been exiled to the margins of politics.[53]

Benner and colleagues emphasize the need for a radical transformation of nursing education that will transform a student into a professional with a capacity for clinical reasoning and critical thinking, who is skilled in patient care, whose practice is self-improving, and who has taken the identity of "nurse" through an educational emphasis on formation and ethical comportment. It appears, however, that the corporatization of higher education, including nursing education, risks pushing nursing education away from formation, away from civic professionalism, and away from both a deeper and broader understanding of human responses to health and illness, pushing instead in the direction of technical professionalism and vocationalism for the sake of a "saleable commodity...a set of workplace skills."[54]

Barrier: Waning of the Liberal Arts

Corporatization, with its emphasis on skill-based, problem-based learning and the reduction of curricular requirements has edged out the liberal arts and the humanities in particular.[55] The second barrier, then, is the reorientation of higher education toward "something more focused and technical" that suppresses the contributions of the liberal arts and humanities.[56] The notion that liberal education is about interesting but superfluous content that may be

---

THINKING ABOUT THINKING AND NURSING EDUCATION...

Courses in logic often begin with an examination of what are called "informal logical fallacies." There are many, not a few of which can be found in political speeches or arguments between parents and adolescents. Many have amusing names: appeal to the stone, proof by verbosity, fallacy of accent, furtive fallacy, gambler's fallacy, homunculus fallacy, Nirvana fallacy, red herring, shotgun argument, and many more. The ancient *trivium*, which formed lower division education, was designed to teach students to spot and dissect these logical fallacies and many more. The *trivium* shaped the student's ability to discover, order, validate, and systematize the facts of reality—what could be discovered through the senses—then to shape them into usable, defensible knowledge. So, basic education was intended to focus intensively on teaching critical thinking (the nursing version of which is the nursing process: assessment, diagnosis, outcomes identification, implementation, and evaluation). After that the student progressed to the *quadrivium*, the second part of the curriculum, as outlined in Plato's *Republic*. Where the *trivium* focused on thought through language, the *quadrivium* focused on thought through numbers—arithmetic, geometry, music and astronomy. Together these formed the liberal arts. The study of the practical arts, like medicine and architecture, could only be undertaken after successful completion of the liberal arts.

As nursing continues to develop, more and more is stuffed into the curriculum which has now come to look like that tall stack of pancakes that no one could possibly eat. The argument is that nursing curriculum is additive—we keep stacking more and more pancakes with removing any—and that content has enlarged at the expense of critical thinking. Nursing students are being given more and more content and skills to prepare them for practice. Yes the students can list the stages of early childhood development and the hallmarks of each stage. But, what do they *think* about child development? Plato wants to know.

---

personally enriching but not occupationally essential is dangerous at several levels. A liberal education teaches habits of mind that impel one toward habits of action. Specifically, liberal learning cultivates broad inquiry for broad understanding, a questioning mind that examines what is contrary to what ought to be, reflective self-understanding and insight, discernment, and cultural participation. Liberal education is essential to understanding the patient holistically, to critical thinking, and to skilled clinical practice. It is equally essential to civic engagement and civic professionalism. Menand notes that

> historical and theoretical knowledge, which is the kind of knowledge that liberal education disseminates, is knowledge that exposes the contingency of present arrangements. ...The goal of teaching students to think for themselves is not an empty sense of self-satisfaction. The goal is to enable students, after they leave college, to make more enlightened contributions to the common good.[57]

The concept of a social contract, theories of professions, critical race theory; intersectionality and race, gender and class; civic professionalism, formation and ethical comportment, culture, and all such interpretations of human life arise from the liberal arts and humanities and are essential the practice of the learned professions—and to nursing.

Historically, the seven liberal arts were the *trivium* (three roads, *vias*, or place where three roads meet) and the *quadrivium* (place where four roads meet). The three subjects of the trivium are language-based and include grammar, logic, and rhetoric. The trivium emphasized critical thinking through input (grammar), process (logic), and output (rhetoric), and comprised lower division education. The four subject matters of the quadrivium then built upon the trivium. They are number-based and include arithmetic (number), geometry (number in space), harmony (music, as number in time), and astronomy (as number in time and space):

> The quadrivium was first formulated and taught by Pythagoras as the *Tetraktys* around 500BC, where all were equal, materially and morally, and where women had equal status to men. It was the first European schooling structure that honed education down to seven essential subjects, later known as the seven liberal arts. ...All these studies offer a safe and reliable ladder to reach the simultaneous values of the True, the Good, and the Beautiful. This in turn leads to the essential harmonious value of Wholeness.[58]

In ancient Greece, the liberal arts were considered essential for the free person (man) to participate in civic life, to defend himself in court, enter into public debate, and otherwise participate in the *polis* or *civitas*. In his 1828 address to the House of Commons, Lord Brougham states that "Education makes a people easy to lead, but difficult to drive; easy to govern, but impossible to enslave."[59] Roth concurs:

> Although Rorty, Nussbaum, and Hirsch have different views of what constitutes liberal learning, they agree that such an education is crucial if we are to have a polity [government] of active citizens rather than passive subjects. The goal, both reflexive and pragmatic, is for students to become independent, autonomous thinkers whose independence and autonomy are enhanced, not compromised, by interaction with others.[60]

Today the liberal arts are interpreted as including both the humanities and the social sciences, though a full liberal education includes the natural sciences as well. The National Endowment for the Humanities (NEH) defines humanities:

> The term 'humanities' includes, but is not limited to, the study and interpretation of the following: language, both modern and classical; linguistics; literature; history; jurisprudence; philosophy; archaeology; comparative religion; ethics; the history, criticism and theory of the arts; those aspects of social sciences which have humanistic content and employ humanistic methods; and the study and application of the humanities to the human environment with particular attention to reflecting our diverse heritage, traditions, and history and to the relevance of the humanities to the current conditions of national life.[61] [According to the NEH], "democracy demands wisdom."[62]

An understanding of the liberal arts is essential to wisdom, to understanding, and to the whole of our lives. Roth makes the point that

> liberal education matters because by challenging the forces of conformity it promises to be relevant to our professional, personal, and political lives. That relevance isn't just about landing one's first job; it emerges over the course of one's working life. The free inquiry and experimentation of a reflexive, pragmatic education help us to think for ourselves, take responsibility for our beliefs and actions, and become better acquainted with own desires, our own hopes. Liberal education matters far beyond the university because it increases our capacity to understand the world, contribute to it, and reshape ourselves. When it works, it never ends.[63]

Barrier: Inacquaintance with Nursing History

The first barrier to education for civic professionalism is the corporatization of higher education (and research), including nursing education. The second is the waning of the liberal arts in favor of a job-ready, technical-skills, vocationalist focus. The third is a lack of knowledge of nursing history. Nursing history is no longer required in most nursing curricula, and it is largely not included even as an elective. Benner and colleagues call for an emphasis on reflective capacity, the meaning and values of nursing, understanding of the changing social context of nursing, history, social sciences, physical sciences, nursing sciences, clinical practice, and ethics, all in the interests of the formation of the student as a nursing professional.[64] It is shortsighted to think that the profession can adequately develop "pride of profession" and "identity" individually or collectively, an understanding of the tradition of meaning and values of nursing, or the social context of nursing, with little or no knowledge of nursing history. We will not dwell on its importance here but the American Association for the History of Nursing offers a position paper providing a rationale for the inclusion of nursing history in all levels of nursing curricula.[65]

Barrier: Educational Entry Point

The fourth, and closely related, barrier of incorporating civic professionalism into nursing education is the multiple educational entry points for nursing. This has been a long, divisive, and painful discussion within the profession and it need not be repeated entirely here, though a few comments are warranted to relate education for entry into practice to education for civic professionalism.

The ANA 1965 position paper "Education for Nursing" called for moving nursing education into institutions of higher education.[66] It called for baccalaureate education as the minimum educational foundation for entry into practice. At the time that the position statement was issued,

> over 85 percent of nurses received their basic education in hospital-sponsored diploma programs; now less than 5 percent do. The percentage of registered nurses receiving training in associate degree programs was less than 2 percent in 1965 but is over 66 percent today. Baccalaureate nursing programs produced about 10 percent of new nurses in 1965, which increased to about a third of new nurses by 1980 and has been stable there for 30 years.[67]

The Institute of Medicine report *The Future of Nursing* recommends that "nurses should achieve higher levels of education and training through an improved education system that promotes seamless academic progression" and that "nurses should be full partners, with physicians and other health professionals, in redesigning health care in the United States."[68] Likewise, *Educating*

Nurses: A Call for Radical Transformation, by Benner and colleagues, calls for the baccalaureate degree as the minimum education for entry into registered nursing practice. Its recommendation is to

> require the BSN [Bachelor of Science in Nursing] for entry to practice. Unlike their colleague educators preparing lawyers, clergy, physicians, and engineers, nursing faculty and preceptors have relatively little time to build a broad and deep knowledge base and guide students in professional formation. Yet nursing requires a high degree of responsibility and judgment in high-risk, underdetermined situations. Thus the baccalaureate degree in nursing should be the minimal educational level for entry into practice. We agree with the Association of American Colleges of Nursing, the American Nursing Association, and other leading nursing organizations that all nursing programs immediately move to baccalaureate degree or master's-level entry for nurses.[69]

Nursing education is central to developing informed civic engagement and civic professionalism. It requires a foundation in liberal education. Nursing has yet to take its place among the learned professions. As Donley and Flaherty note,

> registered nurses…are undereducated members of the health
> care team, when compared with
> physicians, social workers, physical
> therapists, pharmacists, and dieticians to
> name a few. Looking beyond the clinical

THINKING ABOUT EDUCATING GIRLS AND WOMEN...

Higher levels of health and education go hand in hand. While gains have been made in literacy globally, "774 million adults (15 years and older) still cannot read or write—two-thirds of them (493 million) are women. Among youth, 123 million are illiterate of which 76 million are female. Even though the size of the global illiterate population is shrinking, the female proportion has remained virtually steady at 63% to 64%. (See UNESCO's International Literacy Data, 2013: http://www.uis.unesco.org/literacy/Pages/data-release-map-2013.aspx).

It has not always been this way. In ancient Athenian Greece, women and girls were educated and were technically citizens. They could participate in musical competitions, though they could not vote, own land, inherit, defend themselves in court, enter into public discourse, or participate in public life. Well, except for Sparta—there women, like the men, had to do rigorous nude physical training and could drink wine. Historically, however, women have not received the education accorded to men, their writings were much less frequently preserved, and they were legally denied access to institutions of higher education. The movement of nursing from hospital-based diploma programs into institutions of higher education was opposed by many physicians (Nelson, 2002).

---

environment, the nurse work force also lacks the educational credentials of persons in the business, investor, and insurance communities that now play significant roles in health care decisions. *Under-educated members of the health team* rarely sit at policy tables or are invited to participate as members of governing boards. Consequently, there is *little opportunity for the majority of practicing nurses to engage in clinical or health care policy.*[70]

Sullivan and Benner and colleagues identify several educational changes essential to the future of nursing. They include: education for civic professionalism; a foundation in liberal education in order to meet the demand for skilled clinical practice for a widely diverse demographic; a liberal education for engaging in civic professionalism as social activism, social advocacy and more. These essential changes would logically argue for a foundation of liberal education as a bachelor's degree, with a master's degree nursing education built upon it as the entry level for practice. However, for the present, there is another point to be made.

The 1965 position paper "Education for Nursing" was adopted at a time when 85% of nurses in practice were diploma prepared. The profession hitched up its britches, mustered its courage, took a hard line, and threw diploma nurses overboard. In the absence of transition or ladder programs to move diploma nurses to higher levels of education, we (yes, we) were pushed overboard to sink or swim. Diploma programs subsequently closed with astonishing rapidity. It was a wrenching transition for the profession and for diploma nurses who were caught in it. But that change enabled the advance of nursing education, science, and theory to the point that it is beyond question that nursing is a social good essential to the health and well-being of society.

In the field of ethics there is ongoing discussion of the fact–value split. All of the facts in the world will not resolve a value question—they are two different species of question. All the laboratory data, all the diagnostic and prognostic information—clinical certainty even—will not answer the value question of whether it is time to discontinue the ventilator. There is no need for additional facts substantiating better patient outcomes with better-educated nurses, or additional facts substantiating the need to move toward the baccalaureate degree as the minimum educational level for entry into registered nursing practice. It is not a question of fact, it is a question of value and whether nursing has the moral courage it had in 1965 to press forward. BSN entry is not the elephant in the room—it is the stampeding herd of elephants that will crush the profession by division, hurt, continued subordination of nurses in the power dynamics of institutions (amplifying nurses' moral distress), a continued class structure within the profession (inimical to the values of the profession), continued social devaluation of care as "women's work," and a retardation of the progress of its ability to meet the clinical and policy needs of the society that authorizes nursing's existence. As the nursing literature on moral distress[71] and moral courage escalates, it needs to be recognized that, in words of Donley and Flaherty above, nurses are "under-educated members of the health team" and that the educational difference contributes to nurses' lack of opportunity to participate in clinical policy—or to resolve moral distress—in the power dynamics of institutions. Hamric notes that there are "two critical elements of almost every moral distress case: the presence of a power gradient and system issues that complicate the individual patient situation."[72] She characterizes power differentials and the power gradient as alive and well. Diminishing the power differential and lowering the slope of the gradient will require higher levels of nursing education upon entry.

Turner has recently addressed a university audience on moral courage in a presentation entitled "Moral Courage and Ethical Power: The Fearless Heart of Nursing—Feel the Beat."[73] It is long since time for nursing to assert its moral courage and ethical power, to be fearless in moving both the profession and all its individual members forward. In doing so, this time around, it needs to care for those will have to walk the plank by actually helping them swim to a solid landing.

Gedankenexperimente: On the New Economy, Corporatization of Education, and Civic Professionalism

These questions are intended to go beyond the content of the chapter to provoke creative and imaginative thinking about nursing and its social context. The reader might also supply related questions to expand this sample list. Of course, each of these questions could be a separate book.

- In what ways has the new economy affected nursing practice?
- In what way has the corporatization of higher education affected nursing education both for good and for ill?
- What intangible goods does nursing produce?
- Are there ways in which nursing has broken faith with the public?
- Are there ways nursing has failed to keep its social contract?
- What does civic professionalism look like in clinical nursing?
- What if nursing does not transition to BSN entry?
- What if nursing does transition to BSN entry?

- If nursing were to transition to BSN entry, how might it care for those caught in the transition?

- How do multiple entry levels affect nurses in the power dynamics of institutions?

- How do multiple entry levels affect nurses in the power dynamics of professions and society?

- What does nursing as a learned profession look like?

- What is the future of nursing?

ENDNOTES

All URLs provided are accurate as of May 29, 2015.

1   "2012 NAICS," US Census Bureau, North American Industry Classification System, updated May 13, 2013, http://www.census.gov/cgi-bin/sssd/naics/naicsrch?chart=2012.

2   Ibid.

3   "2012 NAICS Definition," US Census Bureau, North American Industry Classification System, updated May 13, 2013, http://www.census.gov/cgi-bin/sssd/naics/naicsrch?chart_code=31&search=2012%20NAICS%20Search.

4   Economic Classification Policy Committee, "Services Classifications," Economic Classification Policy Committee Issues Paper No. 6 (Washington, D.C.: U.S. Department of Commerce, 1993), http://www.census.gov/eos/www/naics/history/docs/issue_paper_6.pdf.

5   "Scope and Standards of Practice,"NursingWorld.org, http://nursingworld.org/scopeandstandardsofpractice.

6   ANA, *Nursing's Social Policy Statement*, 22.

7   Christine Williams, Chandra Miller, and Kristine Kilanski, "Gendered Organizations in the New Economy," *Gender & Society* 26, no. 4 (2012): 549.

8   William Sullivan and Patricia Benner, "Challenges to Professionalism: Work Integrity and the Call to Renew and Strengthen the Social Contract of the Professions," *American Journal of Critical Care* 14, no. 1 (January 2005): 79. Italics in original.

9   William M. Sullivan, *Work and Integrity: The Crisis and Promise of Professionalism in America*. 2nd ed. (San Francisco, CA: Jossey-Bass, 2005), 3, 2.

10   Ibid.

11   M. H. Pappworth, *Human Guinea Pigs: Experimentation on Man* (London: Routledge & Keagan, 1967). See also: Pappworth, "'Human Guinea Pigs'—A History," *British Medical Journal* 301 (December 1990): 1456–60.

12 H. K. Beecher, "Ethics and Clinical Research," *New England Journal of Medicine* 274, no. 24 (June 16, 1966): 1354–60.

13 Fowler, *Guide to the Code of Ethics*, 120.

14 D. Birsch and J. Fielder, *The Ford Pinto Case: A Study in Applied Ethics, Business, and Technology* (Albany: State University of New York Press, 1994).

15 McDonald and Hansen, *Truth, Lies, and O-Rings*.

16 Sullivan and Benner, "Challenges to Professionalism," 78. Italics in original.

17 ANA, *Nursing's Social Policy Statement*, 5.

18 Sullivan, *Work and Integrity*, 5.

19 Ibid. Italics in original.

20 Ibid., 9. Italics in original. See also: Steven Brint, *In An Age of Experts: The Changing Role of Professionals in Politics and Public Life* (Princeton, NJ: Princeton University Press, 1994).

21 Sullivan, *Work and Integrity*, 12.

22 Ibid., 15–18.

23 Ibid., 22.

24 Ibid.

25 Ibid., 23.

26 Ibid.

27 Ibid., 27–30.

28 Ibid., 28.

29 Ibid., 29.

30 Ibid., 32.

31 American Nurses Association, "A Suggested Code," *American Journal of Nursing* 26, no. 8 (August 1926): 599–600.

32 American Nurses Association, "A Tentative Code," *American Journal of Nursing* 40, no. 9 (September 1940): 977.

33 Ibid., 980.

34 American Nurses Association, *A Code for Professional Nurses* [freestanding, one page document] (New York: ANA, 1950).

35 Ibid.

36 American Nurses Association, *Code of Ethics for Nurses with Interpretive Statements* (Washington, DC: ANA, 2001), 29.

37 Ibid., 30.

38 ANA, *Code of Ethics for Nurses* (2001), 30.

39 Harry Boyte and Eric Fretz, "Civic Professionalism," *Journal of Higher Education Outreach and Engagement* 14, no. 2 (2010): 69.

40 ANA, *Code of Ethics for Nurses* (2015), 32.

41 Paragraph adapted from: Fowler, *Guide to the Code of Ethics*, 14.

42 Sullivan, *Work and Integrity*, 195–226.

43 Ibid., 198–99.

44 Ibid., 208.

45 Ibid., 253.

46 Ibid., 253–54.

47 Michael S. Roth, *Beyond the University* (New Haven, CT: Yale University, 2014), 184. See also: Peter John Williams, "Valid Knowledge: The Economy and the Academy," *Chronicle of Higher Education* 54, no. 4 (2007): 511–23.

48 Ellen Schrecker, *The Lost Soul of Higher Education: Corporatization, the Assault on Academic Freedom, and the End of the American University* (New York: The New Press, 2010), 8.

49 Michael Crow, interview by Goldie Blumenstyk, "Knowledge Is a 'Form of Venture Capital' for a Top Columbia Administrator," *Chronicle of Higher Education*, Money & Management Page: A29, http://chronicle.com/article/Knowledge-Is-a-Form-of/17565.

50 Michael Bailey and Des Freedman, *The Assault on Universities: A Manifesto for Resistance* (New York: Palgrave Macmillan, 2011), 146–47. See also: Karen S. Langlois, "A Case Study in University Transformation," *The Journal of Interdisciplinary Studies* 15 (Fall 2002): 49–56.

51 Schrecker, *Lost Soul of Higher Education*, 2.

52 Ibid., 234.

53 Bailey and Freedman, *Assault on Universities*, 2, 145–46. Italics added.

54 Ibid., 151.

55 Schrecker, *Lost Soul of Higher Education*, 163.

56 Fareed Zakaria, *In Defense of a Liberal Education* (New York: W. W. Norton & Company, 2015), 21.

57 Louis Menand, *The Marketplace of Ideas: Reform and Resistance in the American University* (New York: W. W. Norton & Company, 2010), 56.

58 Keith Critchlow, ed., *Quadrivium: The Four Classical Liberal Arts of Number, Geometry, Music, & Cosmology* (New York: Bloomsbury, 2010), 3.

59 Lord Henry Peter Brougham, address to the House of Commons, January 29, 1828; quoted in Angela Partington, ed., Oxford Dictionary of Quotations, 4th ed. (Oxford: Oxford University Press, 1992), 144;, also cited in Victor E. Ferrall Jr., *Liberal Arts At The Brink* (Cambridge, MA: Harvard University Press, 2011), 17.

60 Roth, *Beyond the University*, 180.

61 "About NEH," National Endowment for the Humanities, http://www.neh.gov/about.

62 Ibid.

63 Roth, *Beyond the University*, 195.

64 Patricia Benner et al. *Educating Nurses: A Call for Radical Transformation* (San Francisco: Jossey-Bass/Wiley and Carnegie Foundation for the Advancement of Teaching, 2009).

65 "Position Paper on History in Curriculum," American Association for the History of Nursing, updated September 21, 2001, https://www.aahn.org/position.html.

66 American Nurses Association, "First Position on Education for Nursing," *American Journal of Nursing* 65, no. 12 (December 1965): 106–11.

67 Committee on the Robert Wood Johnson Foundation Initiative on the Future of Nursing, *The Future of Nursing: Leading Change, Advancing Health* (Washington, DC: National Academies Press, 2011), Appendix I, 491.

68 Ibid., 30, 32.

69 Benner, Sutphen, Leonard, and Day, *Educating Nurses*, 216–17.

70 Rosemary Donley and Mary Jean Flaherty, "Revisiting the American Nurses Association's First Position on Education for Nurses," *The Online Journal of Issues in Nursing* 7, no. 2 (May 2002), http://www.nursingworld.org/. MainMenuCategories/ANAMarketplace/ANAPeriodicals/OJIN/TableofContents/ Volume72002/No2May2002/RevisingPostiononEducation.html. Italics added. See also: Timothy G. Smith, "A Policy Perspective on the Entry into Practice Issue," *The Online Journal of Issues in Nursing* 15, no. 1 (October 2009), DOI: 10.3912/OJIN.Vol15No01PPT01; Lucille Joel, "Education for Entry into Nursing Practice: Revisited for the 21st Century," *The Online Journal of Issues in Nursing* 7, no. 2 (May 2002), http://www.nursingworld.org/MainMenuCategories/ ANAMarketplace/ANAPeriodicals/OJIN/TableofContents/Volume72002/ No2May2002/EntryintoNursingPractice.html; Martha A. Nelson, "Education for Professional Nursing Practice: Looking Backward into the Future," *The Online Journal of Issues in Nursing* 7, no. 3 (May 2002), www.nursingworld.org/ MainMenuCategories/ANAMarketplace/ANAPeriodicals/OJIN/TableofContents/ Volume72002/No2May2002/EducationforProfessionalNursingPractice.aspx; and Elizabeth H. Mahaffey "The Relevance of Associate Degree Nursing Education: Past, Present, Future," *The Online Journal of Issues in Nursing* 7, no. 2 (May 2002), www.nursingworld.org/ojin/MainMenuCategories/ANAMarketplace/ ANAPeriodicals/OJIN/TableofContents/Volume72002/No2May2002/ RelevanceofAssociateDegree.aspx.

71 Ann B. Hamric, "A Case Study of Moral Distress," *Journal of Hospice & Palliative Nursing* 16, no. 8 (2014): 457–63. See also: Hamric, "Empirical Research on Moral Distress: Issues, Challenges, and Opportunities," *HEC Forum* 24, no. 1 (March 2012): 39–49; Hamric, "Moral Distress and Nurse-Physician Relationships," *Virtual Mentor* 12, no. 1 (2010): 6–11.

72 Hamric, "Moral Distress and Nurse-Physician Relationships," 4.

73 Martha Turner, "Moral Courage and Ethical Power: The Fearless Heart of Nursing—Feel the Beat," Presentation at the University of Minnesota, March 12, 2015.

Chapter 4.
Nursing: A Covenant of Care

We have moved from an examination of social contract to an examination of what constitutes a profession. From there we looked at what is broken in professions and the need to educate nurses for civic professionalism. Civic professionalism is essential to meeting nursing's social contract. Civic professionalism for nursing is greater than the production of the social good of expert clinical practice; it also extends to institutional change. Nursing has never stopped at the doors of employing institutions. From its early days, nursing has engaged in social criticism and action for social change to affect the health of the whole society. The 1940 *Tentative Code* calls for nurses to work to "promote measures which will advance the interests of humanity."[1] Nursing has stunning historical examples of having done so. But globalization and technological advances make it possible, with great nowness, for nurses to collaborate with other nurses and nursing organizations in an astonishing range of clinical, educational, and research projects around the globe. Nursing seeks the realization of the larger global good of "health for all."

In order to advance the health interests of humanity, nursing must function at the macrolevel, that is, at the political level. Beyond national politics, however, civic professionalism must move beyond the civitas; it must go global—it must be *cosmopolitan*. It is unfortunate that the connotation of cosmopolitan is a person who is sophisticated, stylish, and urbane. The actual denotation, the actual meaning, of cosmopolitan is *citizen of the world*. It derives from the word *cosmopolite* (coś mopolite; kɒzˈmɒpəlaɪt), a compound word, which is both a noun and an adjective. It is constructed from two Greek terms, *kosmos* world + *polites* citizen, thus a world citizen.[2] The nurse–world citizen engages in a form of civic professionalism that goes beyond national boundaries; a *cosmopolite professionalism*.

Like civic professionalism, this form of professionalism requires education and a cognitive apprenticeship. It also requires a sense of calling or vocation, with personal and professional identity and values that are fused. It requires knowledge that seeks wisdom. All of this is rooted in *being*—but what about *doing*? Changing the world for health for all requires that the nurse–cosmopolite professional engage in social ethics with its three functions. Those functions are: reforming one's own profession, asserting the core values of the profession to provoke adherence in the face of competing values, and taking the values of nursing into the social and political arena to bring about change. To do that, nurses collectively, through their professional associations, must analyze both the global power structures and global meaning and value structures. It is through its social ethics and cosmopolite professionalism that nursing serves as a force for health and well-being, and exceeds the demands of social contract. The social contract that authorizes and encompasses nursing is broken, exclusionary, and American. It does not reflect the heroic efforts that modern nursing has made toward national and global health. Nursing exceeds the expectations of its social contract and has extended its relationship with society to that of a social covenant that serves the common good of humanity.

Chapter 1 examined social contract and its critiques. Chapter 2 looked at professions and their role in society. Chapter 3 looked at what is broken in professions and the call for professions to be repaired through civic professionalism, reclaiming a sense of calling, and changing nursing education to include a cognitive apprenticeship with elements of formation and moral comportment. This concluding chapter brings together social contract, professions, and civic professionalism in a way that seeks to repair the brokenness of the social contract. To do this, it considers the critiques of social contract and examines proposed alternatives. It also looks at ways in which cosmopolite professionalism and social covenant can both bring together and extend social contract and civic professionalism.

Educational Formation, Ethical Comportment, and Professional Identity

Sullivan, in *Work and Integrity*,[3] and Benner and colleagues in *Educating Nurses*[4] are calling for a reform of professions, including a reform of nursing.[5] Benner and colleagues regard civic professionalism as an aspect of nurse formation as a professional and at the heart of nursing's social contract.[6] Both Sullivan and Benner and colleagues place heavy weight on the renewal of civic professionalism through educational formation. Benner and colleagues write,

> others call it *socialization*, acquisition of professional values, or development of *professional identity*. We suggest the term *formation* because it denotes development of perceptual abilities, the ability to draw on knowledge and skilled know-how, and a way of being and acting in practice and in the world. …With knowledge and experiential learning, students develop notions of good from their practice

that transform their understanding of nursing's social contract to care for vulnerable patients.[7]

For Sullivan and Benner and colleagues, a part of that formation is teaching and coaching for ethical comportment and the formation of dispositions. These aspects are to be incorporated, with intentionality, into every aspect of nursing education so that "formation occurs as a result of knowledge, skilled know-how, and ethical comportment learned in many concrete situations over time."[8] Over the course of time, the "student moves from *acting* like a nurse to *being* a nurse."[9] Thus, nursing education, as professional education, is a matter of educating for formation of disciplinary knowledge and skill, as well as professional values and identity." These facets are brought together in the 2015 *Code of Ethics for Nurses with Interpretive Statements*. In its discussion of performance standards, it articulates expectations of nursing education:

> Inherent in professional nursing is a process of education and formation. That process involves the ongoing acquisition and development of the knowledge, skills, dispositions, practice experiences, commitment, relational maturity, and personal integrity essential for professional practice. Nurse educators, whether in academics or direct care settings, must ensure that basic competence and commitment to professional standards exist prior to entry into practice.[10]

It is important to note that NSPS addresses the relationship between nursing and society within the social contract, and the reciprocal obligations and expectations of society and nursing. Nursing obligations for competence in practice, as one part of nursing's contractual obligations, are then spelled out in

THINKING ABOUT EDUCATION FOR ETHICAL COMPORTMENT...

Education for formation that includes ethical comportment is not an emphasis that began last Tuesday. Early on, meaning after 1873, the modern nursing education curriculum was understood to include content, skills, and ethics. Its formative elements included inculcating nursing values, fostering citizenship values, and shaping the moral character and dispositions of the student. Essentially, newbie students were moral primordial slime that had to be shaped into moral beings who would bring moral sensibilities and good moral effect both to patient care and to addressing the ills of society by the time they graduated. In 1916 Parsons, in *Nursing Problems and Obligations*, writes "only the character that is built on a foundation of generosity and sweetness (if linked to intelligence, common sense, and humor) is safe in any exigency that may arise. This character foundation is seldom inherited, but must be built up by training and practice" (Parsons, 1916; pg. 8). In recognition of the fact that nurses would practice independently, most often in a patient home, schools of nursing (then called training schools) were about the business of teaching nursing content and skill and engaging in the moral formation of the nursing student. The graduate nurse had to be safe for independent patient care, safe for moral community, and safe for democracy.

the *Nursing: Scope and Standards of Practice*.[11] Nursing's ethical standards, also within the context of nursing's social contract (but also the tradition of nursing) are articulated in the Code.

Formation as Both Doing and Being

However skilled, *acting* like a nurse is not enough. *Being* a nurse is required. There is an interesting distinction that is made in Russian Orthodox theology. It employs three ancient concepts known by their Greek terms: *gnosis, episteme,* and *sophia. Gnosis* is usually translated as "knowledge," though that is a weak translation. Gnosis is knowledge found only in an encounter with another and it is not so much *found* as it is *given.* It is a knowing that includes thought and

---

THINKING ABOUT DOING AND BEING...

The unfortunate Job of the Hebrew Bible would have been a very trying patient. Granted, he was beset by all manner of calamitous misfortune. His sheep were killed in a firestorm, his employees killed by thieves, and a windstorm collapsed his house (killing all his children). Then, Job developed sores from the sole of his foot to the crown of his head. Also, his wife was a harridan. But Job did not endure this with a stiff upper lip. He said,

> I am allotted months of emptiness, and nights of misery are appointed to me. ...my flesh is clothed with worms and dirt; my skin hardens, then breaks out afresh, my days are swifter than a weaver's shuttle and come to their end without hope. Therefore I will not restrain my mouth; I will speak in the anguish of my spirit; I will complain in the bitterness of my soul. (Job 7.3, 5, 6, 11)

Oh no, a complainer! It's going to be a very long shift. However,

> when Job's three friends heard of all these troubles that had come upon him, each of them set out from his home—Eliphaz the Temanite, Bildad the Shuhite, and Zophar the Naamathite. They met together to go and console and comfort him. When they saw him from a distance, they did not recognize him, and they raised their voices and wept aloud; they tore their robes and threw dust in the air upon their heads. They sat with him on the ground seven days and seven nights, and no one spoke a word to him, for they saw that his suffering was very great. (Job 2.11)

Nurses do what needs to be done; they are doers. Let's see: patient Job needs pain meds, antidepressants, rehydration, wound care, marriage counseling, and maybe two of the friends should go to the waiting room? Job's friends got it right. In Job's suffering they came to be with him, just be, not do. Sometimes being is as or more important than doing, and in Job's case it is "being with" or "being in presence." While this is not precisely the same being—doing discussion of the text, it is not unrelated. Being in presence with Job is no therapeutic use of self. It is a way of bringing one's self, one's nursing self, into Job's suffering. Where the nurse has come to the point of being a nurse, where that nursing identity is welded to the nurse's DNA, bringing that nurse-being to the patient's bedside brings together the ontological aspect of nurse-being with an ontological relationship with Job in his suffering. Okay, too much ontology? Bottom line? Sometimes there just are no words to say. It is being together—nurse and Job—that is healing.

(Source: *The New Interpreter's Study Bible NRSV with Apocrypha*. Nashville: Abingdon, 2003.)

---

intellect but is beyond both thought and intellect. Here, in encounter, "thought does not include or seize, but finds itself included and seized."[12] *Episteme,* our second term, is also translated as "knowledge," but it is knowledge of a different sort. It is the knowledge of science and reasoning, emphasizing such things as correlation, causation, analysis and logic, logical relationships, linearity, method, and precision. Episteme must be nourished, informed, and shaped by gnosis, and gnosis by episteme. Both must be held in tension and in balance with one another, for both are important. It is the interpenetration of gnosis and episteme that leads to sophia. *Sophia* is customarily translated as "wisdom." Sophia brings together the two forms of knowledge, forming something new that cannot be achieved by either one alone. It issues into a new way of both doing and being as a skill and should be the goal of cognitive apprenticeship.[13]

Formation that Engages Sophia

The skill expressed in sophia is the skill to adapt one's thought, one's reason, to revelation, to an illumination of the mind and a new way of being, allowing revelation to reconstruct reason and the whole of our faculties of knowing. Picture the musician who plays the piano, a gifted technician of consummate skill, whose playing is perfection itself, but the music is a lifeless technical proficiency. This is episteme. However, in interaction with the audience's responsiveness (encounter), and the inner, perhaps ontological, workings of the pianist (gnosis), both episteme and gnosis come together and produce sophia. We now have a performance that is illuminative, evocative, and soaring, changing both the pianist and the listener. Both the technical knowing (episteme), and the knowing in encounter (gnosis) are essential to each other. As episteme and gnosis meet, the person who once played the piano becomes a pianist— *is* a pianist. This is the nurse whose cognitive apprenticeship is formative. Formation includes both theoretical knowledge and knowledge in encounter, specifically in encounters with those who suffer, are in pain, are anxious, or who are searching for health knowledge. This is the nurse whose formation has prepared a professional with knowledge, skill, compassion, caring, ethical comportment, one who *is* a nurse.[14] This is also a nurse whose formative preparation imbues her or him with a disposition of advocacy. Benner and colleagues note that

> the high expectations for "acting like a nurse" that we saw stressed in nursing programs is a form of civic professionalism (Sullivan, 2005). …Tools for influencing organizational and policy changes are essential, given the current state of health care institutions. Nurses are the ones most present and in a position closest to patients, and their advocacy for improving patient care can be powerful indeed. However, such positive change depends on knowledge and skills to

redesign dangerous and outmoded systems and a unified effort to reduce communication barriers in hierarchical health care systems. To create the level of change needed, partnerships between nurse educators and students in schools of nursing and nursing staff and administrators in service settings are essential. Regulatory bodies for health care institutions and all health care professions need to exert a unified effort at improved collaboration and communication. Each sector must enlarge its boundaries to include all nurses as members and participants in the larger good: effective nursing practice for the sake of a safer and healthier society.[15]

Institutional or societal change is a Sisyphean task. Without the formative changes sought in the cognitive apprenticeship, and without the fusing of professional values to one's identity, there is little to shape one's dispositions and to support perseverance against the odds. Beyond patient care, civic professionalism seeks institutional change. This requires an additional set of organizational and collaborative skills somewhat different from those needed for patient care. These are political skills. These political skills, combined with the social power of the profession through its associations, reaches beyond the institution to the whole of society itself. It reaches even beyond our society to encompass a global citizenship that advocates for global health.

Civic Professionalism Beyond the Bedside

For the remainder of this chapter, civic professionalism will be understood in its activities at the macro level of society, beyond the bedside and the institutional level. We will come to cosmopolite professionalism shortly but first, it is important to explore the dimensions of civic professionalism as it is enacted within our own society. Here, at the heart of civic professionalism are social criticism and social change. More specifically, civic professionalism's civic engagement takes the form of social ethics, as noted in the *Guide to the Code of Ethics*:[16]

> Social ethics is fundamentally about the application of ethics to large, even global, social problems and issues with an emphasis on the sociopolitical conditions and structures that foster injustice. Social ethics may be defined as the domain of ethics that deals with "issues of social order—the good, right, and ought in the organization of human communities and the shaping of social policies. Hence the subject matter of social ethics is moral rightness and goodness in the shaping of human society."[17]

Social ethics engages in social criticism, applying a range of ethical and critical theories that can frame the discussion and move toward policies that will help to redress unjust conditions such as the social determinants of illness, poverty, hunger, illiteracy, and so forth.[18]

The Functions of Social Ethics

There are three fundamental functions of social ethics that are all invoked in civic professionalism: reform of the profession, epideictic discourse (which is a type of public values-based speaking), and social reform.[19,20]

Reform Within

The first function of social ethics—reform of the profession—assures that the profession itself lives up to its own values. Reform seeks to bring the profession and its practice, goals, and aspirations into conformity with the values that it espouses. At times, this necessitates change within the professional community itself, seeking to move the profession toward an envisioned ideal, to bring the "ought" into conformity with the reality of the profession's lived expression. This aspect of social ethics demands intentional, ongoing, critical self-reflection and self-evaluation of the profession based on a range of critical theories that can assist in an incisive, rigorous, self-assessment. For example, it would look at issues of race, gender, and class within nursing, seeking to alleviate any injustices and any harms that are uncovered. Are there issues of racism within the nursing profession?[21] Are there issues of class in nursing?[22] As research on the profession itself uncovers disparities and injustices, small or large, it is morally incumbent upon the profession to do some housekeeping.

Epideictic Discourse

Epideictic discourse, the second function of social ethics, refers to a form of communication that takes place within and for the group. Unfortunately, epideictic has no exact translation in the English language. The term refers to one of Aristotle's three species of rhetoric, specifically to that kind of public speech that reaffirms and reinforces the values that the community itself embraces, especially when confronted with competing values. It "sets out to increase the intensity of adherence to certain values, which might not be contested when considered on their own but may nevertheless not prevail against other values that might come into conflict with them."[23] Epideictic discourse is essentially a rallying cry that reinforces the group's values to the group itself and for the group to others. It strengthens the values that are held in common by the individual members of the group and the speaker, thus "making use of dispositions already present in the audience."[24] Epideictic discourse rallies the troops: it galvanizes the group to employ the group's espoused values in order both to bring about the changes elicited by the first function of social ethics, and to move the group into the third function of social ethics—speaking the values of the group into society at large to help bring about social change that is congruent with the group's values. Epideictic discourse, thus, forms a bridge between the first and second functions of social ethics. It both invokes and evokes the values and dispositions of the members of the group. Examples of epideictic speech in public address abound: Jane Addams's "The Subjective Necessity for Social Settlements"; Susan Anthony's "On Women's Right to Vote"; Eleanor Roosevelt's "The Struggle for Human Rights"; Maya Angelou's "On the Pulse of Morning." The *Suggested Code* of 1926 is another example (remembering that it is now 90 years old):

> Heir throughout the ages of those who have nurtured the young, the weak and the sick, the mother, the kindly neighbor, the knight on the battlefield, the nun and the deaconess within or without enclosing walls—nursing emerges as a profession from its historic setting in an attempt to meet the present demands of society. The most precious possession of this profession is the ideal of service extending even to the sacrifice of life itself.[25]

Social Reform

The third function of social ethics is that of activism in social reform. In this, the profession critiques society, bringing to bear all its social–critical theories. It then attempts to bring about social change that is consistent with the values of the group itself. For instance, if the nursing profession affirms that health is a universal right, which it does in Interpretive Statement 8.1 in *Code of Ethics for Nurses with Interpretive Statements* [26] and that affordable, accessible health care for all is also a right, it would assess the current state of the healthcare system for the following: cost, distribution, and fairness of costs; access and ease of access by all sectors of society, including those with limitations such as mobility, age, literacy, etc., and including ethnic and minority constituencies; and openness of the system to all, including resident noncitizens, tourists, and others. Nursing's value structure emphasizes such values as dignity, health, well-being, caring; thus, nursing would look at healthcare structures for the affirmation of these values as well.

In addition, nursing's assertion of health as a universal right would lead nursing organizations to look at social structures for marks of structural injustice that mitigate against health, that is, the "social determinants of health" and illness. The United Nations notes that

> the bulk of the global burden of disease and the major causes of health inequities, which are found in all countries, arise from the conditions in which people are born, grow, live, work and age. These conditions are referred to as social determinants of health, a

term used as shorthand to encompass the social, economic, political, cultural and environmental determinants of health.[27]

Nursing research, scholarship, policy, and activism in social, economic, political, cultural, and environmental spheres is essential if nursing is to be involved in seeking to ameliorate structurally caused inequities in health. It requires social ethics and is therefore an intrinsically social and political engagement that is the work of nursing professional associations, in part through their political action committees.

It is expected that all nurses will be involved in some way in this aspect of the profession's social ethics. This involvement requires acquiring knowledge about social conditions, informed voting, and participation in legislative processes through local and national representatives. For some it will involve research or policy formation. While individuals do not themselves bring about major social change, they may lead it. These leaders will have a movement that forms behind them. While some charismatic nursing leaders are able to lead social change as individuals, the actual implementation of social criticism and social change, and momentum for change, depends upon collective action, usually through a professional association. In order to engage in social criticism and to bring about social change, the profession must have knowledge based in critical theories that can guide and deepen social analysis and critique. Critical theories have different perspectives but hold in common that they are explanatory, practical, and normative (ethical). Here a range of theories are used to both critique society (and the profession itself). Postcolonial, feminist, liberation, Marxist, and critical race theories are examples. Not unlike the structure of the nursing process, the goal of these theories is to uncover, explain, plan, and act to transform social conditions "to liberate human beings from the circumstances that enslave them."[28]

Nurses now need to know how to shape health policy—now, not in some distant future. The IOM report *The Future of Nursing: Leading Change, Advancing Health* calls upon nurses to take an active part in shaping policy. It states:

> Being a full partner [in health care] translates more broadly to the health policy arena. To be effective in reconceptualized roles, nurses must see policy as something they can shape rather than something that happens to them. Nurses should have a voice in health policy and be engaged in implementation efforts related to health care reform. Nurses also should serve actively on advisory committees, commissions, and boards where policy decisions are made to advance health systems to improve patient care.[29]

Cognitive Apprenticeship for Political Involvement

In order to bring about social change that liberates, these theories and knowledge of political and policy processes becomes essential. The resources of the professional association, including its political action committees (PACs), would then be drawn upon to support action for social change. It is important to this function of the profession's social ethics that nurse educators include in nursing curricula content on social ethics relating to issues of justice, social theories, nursing history related to social involvement of nursing and nurses, health policy formulation, and the state and federal political processes. As importantly, Sullivan and Benner and colleagues call for a cognitive apprenticeship, with its three facets, for developing civic professionalism for nursing practice in nursing education. That same cognitive apprenticeship is essential to developing social and political analysts and activists within the profession. There is a range of opportunities both for students and for graduates to assist in developing these skills. The American Association of Colleges of Nursing offers the Government Affairs Internship, as do a number of universities, the IOM, the Robert Wood Johnson Foundation, the Hartford Foundation, and others.[30] However, in addition to these special opportunities, cultural, social, and political analysis should be a part of all nursing education.

As noted in the previous chapter, Sullivan and Benner and colleagues have called for cognitive apprenticeships that are comprised of three components: (a) intellectual or cognitive apprenticeship as found in the university context, (b) "imagined or simulated practice situations" taught by competent practitioners, and (c) an introduction of students to "the values and attitudes shared by the professional community" by teaching "the skills and traits, along with the ethical comportment, social roles, and responsibilities that mark the professional."[31] This last component, rooted in both values and a disposition to action helps to prepare nurses in good measure both for civic professionalism and for the first two functions of social ethics (reform within and epidictic discourse). By including a stronger emphasis on critical theories and policy in the baccalaureate and graduate levels of nursing education, and by creating and incorporating social ethics-cognitive apprenticeships available with politically and legislatively active nurse leaders, nurses will be better prepared to move into social criticism and social change, specifically into social and political civic professionalism. However, nursing activism must go beyond national borders.

Globalization

Globalization has shrunk the world. Nurse scholars collaborate transnationally, nurse researchers conduct research in international venues, nursing schools offer opportunities for education abroad. International communication, collaboration, education research, and of course migration, have become commonplace. UNESCO does not land on a single definition of globalization but indicates its attributes:

> There are many suggestions and debates on the question of how to define the concept of globalisation. Here are some few definitions commonly used:
>
> *Globalisation is a multi-dimensional process characterised by:*
>
> - The acceptance of a set of economic rules for the entire world designed to maximise profits and productivity by universalising markets and production, and to obtain the support of the state with a view to making the national economy more productive and competitive;
>
> - technological innovation and organisational change centred on flexi-bilisation and adaptability; the expansion of a specific form of social organisation based on information as the main source of productivity and power;
>
> - the reduction of the welfare state, privatisation of social services, flexibilisation of labour relations and weaker trade unions;
>
> - de facto transfer to trans-national organisations of the control of national economic policy instruments, such as monetary policy, interest rates and fiscal policy;
>
> - the dissemination of common cultural values, but also the re-emergence of nationalism, cultural conflict and social movements.[32]

We must note here, in passing, that globalization is fundamentally economic in nature. Globalization means that nurses can no longer be stay-at-home nurses or stay-at-home civic professionals. Nurses must, instead, be or become global citizens as persons and cosmopolite professionals as nurses. The UNESCO document *Education for 'Global Citizenship'* points out that

> the multiple processes of globalization—whether economic, technological, environmental, or political—are progressively transforming traditional conceptions and practices of citizenship. The consolidation of the international human rights regime, the greater interconnectedness and interdependence of individuals and groups across the world, and the emergence of new forms of transnational or post-national civic engagement are all expressions of this transformation.[33]

Global Citizenship and Cosmopolitanism

The concept of global citizenship is not without problems. It is a metaphor—as a legal concept it has no validity, as one cannot be a citizen of the world in any legal sense. UNESCO acknowledges Falk, who "had proposed categories of 'global citizens' which included transnational and global activists, or an emerging 'cosmopolitan community of individuals' which was seen as expressing new forms of post-national citizenship."[34] The claim is that

> globalization, and the growing acknowledgement that individuals around the world are increasingly, directly and indirectly, interconnected and interdependent beyond the local communities and nation-states to which they belong, is making cosmopolitanism not only a reality, but a necessity.[35] Cosmopolitanism is based on an acknowledgement of the legitimacy of the principle of universality. Indeed, the principle of universality is fundamental to humanist, humanitarian, and human rights perspectives where, in addition to being members of local communities and citizens of nation-states, individuals are also seen as members of a *global* community of human beings.[36]

UNESCO prefers cosmopolitanism to global citizenship because of contested notions of what constitutes citizenship:

> The articulation of local/national and global realities affecting citizenship are making cosmopolitanism all the more relevant in the early 21st century: cosmopolitanism that is based on the principles of diversity/difference in universality. Rather than the potentially contested notion of "global citizenship education', it may perhaps be more appropriate to refer to education for 'cosmopolitan citizenship', or to citizenship education in a global world.[37]

The UNESCO recommendations for education for cosmopolitan citizenship identify four key thematic areas: Human rights, environmental issues, issues of social and economic justice, and intercultural issues.[38] These recommendations pertain to all education, for every person, in every nation. They are not recommendations specific to nursing education, or any specific profession for that matter. In fact, the recommendations are actually intended for primary and secondary education, directed toward all young persons.

Cosmopolite Professionalism

Our concern here is not for a universal cosmopolitanism but instead for how that should be incorporated in the nursing professional role. All nurses should be citizens of the world, but what does that mean for nursing as cosmopolite professionals?

One will find ample research and scholarship in the nursing literature in each of the four thematic issues UNESCO identifies. To the question of who decides what is to be included in cosmopolitan citizenship education in nursing, the response is: the long tradition of modern nursing that has and continues to wrestle with these concerns. The UNESCO concern is that all persons be or become cosmopolitan citizens whose education seeks to produce awareness of the wider world and a sense of own role both as a citizen with rights and responsibilities, and as a member of the global human community. UNESCO identifies four thematic issues:

- Valuation of the diversity of cultures and of their languages, arts, religions, and philosophies as components the common heritage of humanity.

- Commitment to sustainable development and sense of environmental responsibility.

- Commitment to social justice and sense of social responsibility.

- Willingness to challenge injustice, discrimination, inequality and exclusion at the local/national and global level in order to make the world a more just place[39]

However, if a nurse is to have both knowledge and skills as well as a "willingness to challenge injustice, discrimination, inequality and exclusion at the local/national and global level in order to make the world a more just place" it requires the cognitive apprenticeship that Sullivan calls for. Here that cognitive apprenticeship is for addressing the global issues that affect health. To do so necessitates employing the third function of social ethics, the engagement with social criticism and social change. Social criticism for social change begins with an examination of two types of social structures: global power structures and global meaning and value structures.

Meaning and Value Structures and Power Structures

Fundamentally, engaging in social criticism and social change involves an analysis of both the meaning and value structures, and the power structures that surround an issue. Meaning and value structures are all those professional structures that embed, carry, and implement the values of a group. For example, for nurses, the meaning and value structures include national and international codes of ethics for nurses, the values and ethics literature of the profession, the moral motifs of the profession (e.g., service, caring), the explicit ends of the profession (e.g., health, dignity, well-being) as articulated in position statements and documents, international human rights and human protections policies or statements, humanitarian goals of the profession, and more. The meaning and value structures of a profession guide and inform, and in some cases, critique and limit the action of a profession. More specifically, the meaning and value structures of a profession are held in balance with its power structures. Power structures include any and all sources of social and political power, including social prestige, autonomy of the profession, money, and authority. It is a profession's power structures (e.g., nursing associations, PACs, unions, accrediting bodies, etc.) that make things happen, that bring about the realization of the meaning and power structures. Without power structures, meaning and value structures are impotent. Power structures must be used to implement meaning and value structure ends, as it is a profession's meaning and value structures that prevent runaway self-interest of a profession, prevent its abuse of authority, and generally identify lines that should never be crossed. When a profession breaks faith with the public and is in breach of the social contract, it is because the power structures overwhelmed the meaning and value structures and the meaning and value structures could not contain the power structures. Such is the case in the examples in Chapter 2.

Any attempt to affect global health, global health disparities, pandemics and other health concerns will need to investigate global power structures that have become root causes or contributors. These include commerce and trade, economics, politics, culture, religion, government—in short, all of the

---

THINKING ABOUT POWER STRUCTURES...

The king of Egypt, called Pharaoh, ruled a 13th century BC empire and oppressed its Hebrew slaves horribly. He feared their growing numbers so he summoned the Hebrew midwives to command them.

> The king of Egypt said to the Hebrew midwives, one of whom was named Shiphrah and the other Puah, "When you act as midwives to the Hebrew women, and see them on the birthstool, if it is a boy, kill him; but if it is a girl, she shall live." But the midwives feared God; they did not do as the king of Egypt commanded them, but they let the boys live. So the king of Egypt summoned the midwives and said to them, "Why have you done this, and allowed the boys to live?" The midwives said to Pharaoh, "Because the Hebrew women are not like the Egyptian women; for they are vigorous and give birth before the midwife comes to them." (Exodus 1.15-20)

Yeah, right. Ethnicity makes a difference in birthing physiology? But then, what do kings know about birthing? The midwives did not exactly "speak truth to power." They outright lied, and put their lives at risk for the well-being of birthing mothers and their male neonates. They lied. And, midwives refused to participate in Nazi experiments or in Beecher's 22 unethical research projects.

(Source: *The New Interpreter's Study Bible NRSV with Apocrypha*. Nashville: Abingdon, 2003.)

---

macro-affectors of life. The global meaning and value structures include the wide range of human rights agreements, a range of international accords, a wide range of U.N. documents, including the supporting documents and agreements for each of the U.N. Millennium Development Goals, the UNESCO document *Global Citizenship Education*,[40] and the World Health Organization, World Medical Association, and International Council of Nurses documents, codes of ethics, and policy statements. In addition, there are cultural and religious meaning and values resources. (We will not pause here to provide a specific example; that will follow in the Afterword.)

There is always the question of "Where to begin?" The profession as a whole, through its associations may work on several fronts simultaneously. But an individual nurse will need to choose a target issue for which she or he has a passion that will sustain activism when the going is tough or seemingly refractory to change. Civic professionalism may even manifest as marshaling nurses to political activism, independent of a specific issue. As to specific issues, engaging civic professionalism for national health finds a ready menu of issues to address in the multiple Institute of Medicine Reports. The issues they contain are wide ranging and include diversity and disparity in health care, health literacy, transforming the work environment for nurses, preventing childhood obesity, pre-term births, and a host of other concerns, most having connections to issues of race, class, ethnicity, and gender.[41] To identify issues of global concern, one need only look to the U.N. Millennial Development Goals with their specific targets, and such agreements as the 1978 *Declaration of Alma Ata* where the phrase "Health for All by the year" was coined.[42] The U.N. Millennium Goals are:

Goal 1: Eradicate extreme poverty and hunger

Goal 2: Achieve universal primary education

Goal 3: Promote gender equality and empower women

Goal 4: Reduce child mortality rates

Goal 5: Improve maternal health

Goal 6: Combat HIV/AIDS, malaria, and other diseases

Goal 7: Ensure environmental sustainability

Goal 8: Develop a global partnership for development[43]

Each goal has several specific targets, any one of which can be a focus of individual or collective effort in accord with the passions, interests, and skills of the nurse or organization. With the diversity of specialized nursing organizations, these Millennium Development Goals could be attacked at several points.

A united and coordinated effort by nursing organizations could be a powerful instrument for global change.

There has been a rising interest in nursing for health diplomacy, and health diplomacy is one means for nursing to enact cosmopolite professionalism. In the international arena, health must compete with all other goods, such as commerce, military, and education expenditures. Health diplomacy works to bring health concerns into parity with competing values. Health must not continue to fall to the bottom of the pile; health diplomacy seeks to turn this around. Citing Koplan, Hunter and colleagues define health diplomacy:

> The term global health refers to "an area for study, research, and practice that places a priority on improving health and achieving equity in health for all people worldwide. Global health emphasizes trans-national health issues, determinants, and solutions; involves many disciplines within and beyond the health sciences and promotes interdisciplinary collaboration; and [it] is a synthesis of population based prevention with individual-level clinical care."[44]

We must move now from the concerns of global health to a reconsideration of the adequacy of social contract as a framework for nursing's national and global engagement.

The Adequacy of Social Contract as a Framework

A social contract is a fairly minimalistic social arrangement. In exchange for professions' control of their work, architects' buildings should not fall down, dentists' fillings should not fall out, physicians' patients should not be harmed, and clergy should pray, not prey. The expectations of the social contract are minimum expectations below which no profession should fall. The contract does not demand excellence, or that professions go beyond its demands. In addition, as was noted in the first chapter, there are a number of concerns for the adequacy of social contract. To recap, the concerns are as follows.

> *The social contract is exclusionary:* The social contract itself is broken in terms of race, ethnicity, gender, class, and disability. Social contract is a part of the power structure, not the meaning and value structure, and the social arrangements that it structures are damaging and disadvantaging to women and minority subgroups of society.

> *The social contract devalues care work:* Even in a service society, technologically based services are valued, while care services and woman-dominant occupations remain disvalues.

The social contract is, at base, rooted in economic and protectionist concerns:
To return to Rousseau, "it should be remembered that the foundation of the social compact is property; and its first condition, that everyone should be maintained in the peaceful possession of what belongs to him."[45] Recalling the discussion of the first chapter, the development of a concept of private property is attended by the development of greed, competition, and other vices, in addition to inequality, social classes, and ultimately warfare,[46] problems that will be taken up shortly.

A range of critiques of social contract have emerged, each proposing an approach that will remedy a failing of social contract. We will look particularly at the work of Nussbaum and Tronto, two approaches that are congenial to nursing.

Nussbaum's Capabilities Approach

Nussbaum's *Capabilities Approach* works on the issue of the exclusionary nature of the social contract. More specifically, she critiques the chain of social contract theories, including its more recent development in the work of John Rawls. Nussbaum's critique is extended, nuanced, and thorough and the reader is invited to examine her works.[47] Rawls's reformulation of social contract has unresolved problem areas that Rawls himself acknowledges: justice across national lines; the fair treatment of people with disabilities; and the moral treatment of nonhuman animals. She formulates her theory so that it addresses Rawl's three problem areas; she does not seek to replace either Rawls or social contract theory, but rather to reenvision the contract itself to be more inclusive. Nussbaum admits that the "Capabilities Approach has not been shown to be superior to Rawls's version of the social contract in all areas—only in these three problem areas."[48] Nussbaum holds that "all contract theories, including Rawls's, assume a rough equality of physical and mental power among the participants"[49] and that

> the assumptions of rough equality and mutual advantage mean that
> [it] cannot deal well with cases in which we find a deep asymmetry
> of power between the parties that is not easily corrected by simply
> rearranging income and wealth. Precisely for that reason, people
> with severe physical and cognitive disabilities are explicitly omitted
> from the Original Position and are not included under the definition
> of the capacities of citizens in the Well Ordered Society. Their needs,
> says Rawls, are to be dealt with at some point but are not taken into
> account when society selects its most basic principles and structures.
> In effect, they are to be dominated, though the domination is to
> be beneficent. This problem is exacerbated by the fact that Rawls's

Kantian conception of the person is based on rationality (both pru-
dential and moral): so people with severe cognitive disabilities just
don't count as persons under that view. Rawls explicitly holds that
human beings who can't enter into agreements or contracts are not
owed political justice. Thus for Rawls the whole issue of justice is
moot for at least many people with disabilities.[50]

She makes the point that social contract theory "maintains that the contract
is to the mutual advantage of the participants; it is advantage, not altruism or
love of others, that brings them together in society."[51] This is a point that we
will need to pick up later. Her intent is that national and international development priorities be human development and that human development not
be lost to economic growth (the very problem that we see with the structural
adjustment policies that are discussed in the case in the Afterward). As an
alternative approach to development economics, the Capabilities Approach

begins from a commitment to the equal dignity of all human beings,
whatever their class, religion, caste, race, or gender, and it is committed to the attainment, for all, of lives that are worthy of that
equal dignity. Both a comparative account of the quality of life and
a theory of basic social justice, it remedies the major deficiencies of
the dominant approaches. It is sensitive to distribution, focusing particularly on the struggles of traditionally excluded or marginalized
groups. It is sensitive to the complexity and the qualitative diversity
of the goals that people pursue. Rather than trying to squeeze all
these diverse goals into a single box, it carefully examines the relationships among them, thinking about how they support and com-
plement one another. It also takes account of the fact that people
may need different quantities of resources if they are to come up to
the same level of ability to choose and act, particularly if they begin
from different social positions.[52]

Tronto's Political Ethic of Care

Among all the theorists of an ethic of care, Tronto's approach comes closest to
an actual political theory. She looks specifically at intersections of gender, race,
class, care ethics, feminist theory, and political science. Tronto addresses the
marginalization and devaluation of care work and its relegation to the private
sphere. She identifies three "moral boundaries" that erect barriers between
ethics and politics and that have obstructed an ethic of care. These boundaries
are: (a) the separation of morality and politics, (b) the abstraction of morality,
and (c) the separation of the public and private sphere.[53] While an ethic of care
has been relegated, generally, to a "women's morality," Tronto demonstrates

that it has a close affinity with the 18th-century Scottish Enlightenment, when these boundaries did not exist. She proceeds to show that these three moral boundaries are a social construction arising within the social transformations of the 18th century, and that these boundaries need not prevail.[54]

Tronto claims "the practice of care is a political ideal"[55]; she seeks to bring care in as a core political value and as a political vision. Her claim is that care is essential to democracy and that

> to include the value of caring in addition to commitments to other liberal values (such as a commitment to people's rights, to due process, to obeying laws and following agreed-upon political procedures) makes citizens more thoughtful, more attentive to the needs of others, and therefore better democratic citizens.[56]

In the face of the three boundaries, embracing an ethic of care would require that we reconceptualize our moral understandings. We would need to acknowledge that Kantian autonomy is a fiction; that no one is fully autonomous, we are all interdependent. Second, we would have to acknowledge that all persons need care, that at times our lives range between independence and dependence in varying degrees and that dependence is a part of the human condition. There would also need to be a shift from a focus on *interests* (as in self-interest) to *needs*. An ideal of *moral detachment* (as in the dispassionate and disinterested moral decision-maker) would need to be overturned in favor of *moral engagement*. The fiction of human equality would need to be overtaken by recognition of that equality as a goal, and that some will need additional resources to reach equality. Care activities, even if continued in the private sphere, would count as citizen activities. And finally, we would have to acknowledge that "justice without care is incomplete."[57] These movements fundamentally reorient ethics, changing its moral boundaries. While Tronto's concern is largely national, democratic citizenship, she does not limit an ethic of care to the American polity. Her four elements of an ethic of care in practice (attentiveness, responsibility, competence, and responsiveness) are sufficiently broad to permit cultural variation in understanding and implementation. Tronto's ethic of care, in effect, causes meaning and value structures to interpenetrate power structures.

Toward a More Adequate Framework

At its base, a social contract is a protectionist social arrangement: society is protected from professions and professions are protected from society's encroachment. It is a contract of mutual advantage, as Nussbaum notes, so that parties are expected to meet its requirements, but nothing more. Social contract is driven by "mutual advantage," not altruism or love, as Nussbaum notes. In addition, the issue of private property is the bedrock of social contract. It is essential to recall the words from the first chapter:

> The development of a concept of private property (my land, my plow, my pickaxe, etc.) follows, and with it the development of greed, competition, vanity, deceit, and a host of vices, in addition to inequality, social classes, and ultimately warfare; "in short," Rousseau writes, "competition and rivalry on the one hand, opposition of interests on the other, and always the hidden desire to profit at the expense of someone else. All these ills are the first effect of property and the inseparable offshoot of incipient inequality."[58] It is private property that is pivotal in making civil society and government necessary. Those who have property want government to protect their property, to advantage them, and to cement inequality. In Rousseau's opinion, it is also private property for which "the vices that make social institutions necessary are the same ones that make their abuses inevitable."[59]

This was Rousseau's social contract gone wrong, not his corrective formulation that had built in safeguards against exploitation, inequality, greed, and a host of vices. Yet this is exactly what is seen today, as in the Enron, banking, and Wall Street scandals, labor exploitation globally, and in the professions breaking faith with the public and breaching their social contracts. That said, social contract is here to stay; it is embedded in the US Constitution and the American national character. It may be able to be made more inclusive of persons, caring, and more if globalization can be directed toward the ends of health as well.

Nursing and Supererogation

Social contract authorizes the existence of nursing and its practice, and yet it is no mirror of the tradition and essence of nursing, which demonstrates altruism, caring, and even love of humanity, rather than operating solely on terms of mutual benefit. Modern nursing has a long history of civic professionalism, cosmopolite professionalism, altruism and supererogation, a concern for the common good, and more. *Supererogation* is the ethical term for acts that go beyond what is required, beyond the call of duty. Discussions of supererogation have largely been found in the theological literature, especially Thomas Aquinas's *Summa Theologica*, works by Luther and Calvin,[60] and Maimonides on *lifnim mi'shurat ha'din* (beyond the line of the law).[61] Urmson's 1958 article "Saints and Heroes" initiates the discussion of supererogation in the modern philosophical literature.[62] There are well-known examples of supererogation in nursing's history. Clara Maass is one such example. She was a volunteer contract nurse during the Spanish American war (when nurses could not be members of the military), was discharged and volunteered again to serve in the Philippines. In Cuba, she volunteered to participate in an investigation of yellow fever. She volunteered to be bitten by mosquitos carrying yellow fever, contracted yellow fever, recovered, volunteered to be bitten again, and died of the illness.[63] The US postage stamp honoring her states "She gave her life." There are, however, thousands of nurses who have died in service, whose work was supererogatory. For example, over 10,000 US nurses served in France during World War I: "Many, however, who went into service did not return. On the Service Flag hanging at National Headquarters of the American Red Cross, 261 gold stars appear."[64] The stars represent the 261 American Nurses who died in service in France. Nurses who have served during wars have been volunteer, civilian, and contract nurses, as well as (after 1901) military nurses. Women were not drafted; they volunteered to serve in the military. Other nurses, not serving in the military or conflict zones, have died in service. These largely unnamed nurses cared for patients during epidemics (e.g., influenza, yellow fever, typhus) and natural disasters and were termed *victimes du devoir* (victims of duty) or *victimes de leur dévouement* (victims of their devotion). Supererogation does not necessarily lead to death; the sacrifice of life for another is at the outer edge of supererogation. It seems unlikely that there would be any nurse who could not find personal examples in her or his own life or that of colleagues who went the second mile, went beyond duty in nursing care, who demonstrated altruism, caring, and a love of humanity that exceeded the demands of the social contract.

Nursing and Self-Interest

Nursing has also been remarkably balanced in its concern that the wages of nurses not be secured to the detriment of patients. As previously noted, service, not pecuniary self-interest, has been and remains an ideal of the profession. This has not prevented nurses from actively seeking just compensation and doing so by what it considers just means. An examination of the nursing discourse on strikes, work stoppages, unions, and collective bargaining is a good starting point for exploring nursing's concern to balance competing interests, but beyond the scope of this work.

Nursing and the Common Good

Nursing also demonstrates a profound concern for the common good. *Common good* is a difficult concept to define. "I know it when I see it" (a phrase made famous by Supreme Court Justice Stewart in reference to a threshold for "obscenity" in film) is how most approach defining the common good.[65] But we need to provide some refinement of the concept.

The common good does not happen on its own; it has to be brought about intentionally. The common good consists in having all the social structures, specifically the power structures, that we rely upon work together in ways such that everyone is included and everyone benefits. The content of the common good is historically and culturally contingent so that in different time periods and in different cultures it will be defined differently. Some examples of goods that are a part of the common good in the contemporary United States include health care, road maintenance, fire protection, and education. When these social structures do not work properly, social problems arise, such as inequitable access to health care, better road maintenance and fire protection in wealthier communities, differences in the quality of education available and in general, the kinds of issues of race, gender, class, ethnicity and ability that were indicated earlier. Each person should do what he or she can to contribute to the common good, but the "free-rider problem" is often mentioned in terms of the common good.

The free-rider is the person who enjoys the benefits of the common good but does not contribute to it. This points to a tension that exists in American society. The culture values "rugged individualism" and our culturally attenuated ethics give priority to autonomy and respect for autonomy. The person who chooses not to participate in the common good but rather to pursue self-interest is at odds with the very concept of the common good. Beerbohn and Davis note these and other difficulties with the concept of the common good. In the end they advance what they call a "buck-passing account" of the common good by defining it as "The *Buck-Passing Account of the Common Good:* Being in the common good consists in the fact that there are reasons to act together to bring it about."[66]

The common good is a concept widely embraced and discussed in Catholic Social Teachings. The Vatican decree *Gaudium et Spes* examines humanity's relationship to society and the human community, and includes statements on issues of wealth, resources, and economics, poverty, social justice, and culture, and science and technology. The decree states that

> every day human interdependence grows more tightly drawn and spreads by degrees over the whole world. As a result the common good, that is, *the sum of those conditions of social life which allow social groups and their individual members relatively thorough and ready access to their own fulfillment*, today takes on an increasingly universal complexion and consequently involves rights and duties with respect to the whole human race. Every social group must take account of the needs and legitimate aspirations of other groups, and even of the general welfare of the entire human family.[67]

In a less stilted more understandable English, the common good is "the whole network of social conditions which enable human individuals and groups to flourish and live a fully, genuinely human life, otherwise described as 'integral human development.'"[68] Values central to this understanding of the common good include human dignity, solidarity, human freedom with responsibility, democracy, human rights, equality, the right to property, the social responsibility of companies, the alleviation of poverty, and care for the poor. There is a concern for many social structures and conditions that affect the common good, including a particular concern for the poor:

> If any section of the population is in fact excluded from participation in the life of the community, even at a minimal level, then that is a contradiction to the concept of the common good and calls for rectification. If that exclusion comes about from poverty, even if only "relative poverty", then that poverty demands attention. Governments cannot be satisfied with provision for poor people designed only to prevent absolute poverty, such as actual starvation or physical homelessness.[69]

All the major formulations of the common good hold that it is only truly realized within the context of a democracy. They also affirm a right of property ownership, commerce, the formation of corporations, and more. The Vatican decree on the common good, and many other discussions of the common good, specifically deny that the common good can be achieved in totalitarian, oligarchic, autocratic governments. Dictatorships, even benevolent dictatorships, and the common good simply do not go together.

However, the common good can bump up against self-interest. It is not so much pitted against self-interest per se, as against inordinate self-interest that undermines, or damages the common good, or overrides and excludes other human values. Self-interest itself is not cast as wrong but as a normal feature of the human condition, rooted in survival. It is self-interest to the harm of others that comes under criticism. Discussions of the 99% and the 1% in the distribution of wealth become, at some point, discussions of the common good versus self-interest. Globalization is characterized, with good reason, as the corporatization of the world that has ignored the common good to enrich the few. There is an emerging literature, however, that asserts that "it is likely that the business sphere will not be in a position to disregard the global common good much longer."[70] Bettignies and Lépineux claim that there are "three major determining factors that are likely to drive corporations to take the global common good into account: the deterioration of the biosphere, the rise of an anti-globalization sentiment, and the necessity to invent a global social contract."[71]

From Social Contract to Social Covenant

The challenges posed by the global economic recession have caused global institutions to renew their efforts to address increasing poverty and hunger, conflict migrations, and a host of world social conditions that are constantly in the headlines. The World Economic Forum (WEF), a prestigious, influential, independent, and non-partisan international institution, focuses its concern on an astonishing range of global issues covered by its many expert councils. Founded in 1971, the WEF is a membership organization comprised of "1,000 of the world's top corporations, global enterprises usually with more than US$ 5 billion in turnover. These enterprises rank among the top companies within their industry and play a leading role in shaping the future of their industry and region."[72] WEF's Global Agenda Council on Values asks "how can we ensure that human dignity and common values are at the centre of economic pursuits?"[73] Its answer is, in part, to construct "The Moral Economy: From Social Contract to Social Covenant." WEF calls for a "new social covenant." In their cover letter they write the following:

> The world is facing a series of difficult challenges and adjustments:
> We face a broken social contract and declining social trust in developed economies. There are very difficult choices that come with austerity and retrenchment. We see serious resource mal-distribution and constraints; and experience growing conflicts. The need for equitable growth in developing nations is clear; and the need for a moral agenda to overcome extreme poverty. ...So this is our call: for a period of intentional, global reflection on the values we bring to

---

THINKING ABOUT COVENANT...

There is nothing intrinsically wrong with contracts. They are very useful legal agreements that keep transactions orderly. Party A does this and Party B does that. Both this and that are specified precisely. Party A and B neither fall below nor go beyond the contract's provisions. If one party does not meet the stipulations of the contract, the other can take legal action. It's clean, it's simple...it's minimal. In a contractual arrangement, one need not be a good person, one only need meet the conditions of the contract. While it is a contractual relationship, it is not much of a relationship. Some relationships are not meant to be contractual:

Spouse A: I will take the trash out if you do the laundry.
Spouse B: I will do the laundry, but only one load of wash since that's what taking out the trash is worth. And you will have to dry and fold it yourself.

In this contract there is no: "I see that you are tired. You should just relax take it easy. I will take the trash out, do the laundry, and run you a hot bath."

Covenantal relationships offer something that contracts cannot. They embrace human relatedness, are rooted in authentic relationship, are responsive to the need of the other, give when there can be no take; presume goodwill, generosity, and trust; expect goodness, and seek the good for all.

---

the largest decisions of our time. A method to foster that reflection is the development of a New Social Covenant. There is great cultural diversity when it comes to values. But there is also a broad consensus—across cultures, religions and philosophies—on some shared, human aspirations.

- The dignity of the human person—whatever their race, gender, background or belief.

- The importance of a common good that transcends individual interests.

- The need for stewardship—a concern, not just for ourselves, but for posterity.

Together these offer a powerful, unifying ideal: Valued individuals, committed to one another, and respectful of future generations.[74]

WEF's concern is for responsible corporate behavior and globalization that sustains and even furthers the common good while still affirming global trade and commerce. WEF proposes a twofold move that will support a list of values and ends that they affirm and will serve to ameliorate social inequality and restore social trust. The first is the movement from a shareholder to a stakeholder economy and the second is the creation of a social covenant to replace social contract. To move from a shareholder economy to a stakeholder economy means to move "from a narrowly defined shareholder economy to a stakeholder economy that includes workers, consumers, rights advocates, the environment, and future generations—all in our economic calculations and decision-making."[75] The WEF report continues:

> The collapse of financial systems and resulting economic crises has generated a growing disbelief and a fundamental distrust in the ways things operate and how decisions are made. Old social contracts have unraveled. Former assumptions and shared notions about fairness, agreements, reciprocity, mutual benefits, social values, and expected futures have all but disappeared. …Over the last 20 to 30 years, we have witnessed a massive breakdown in trust between citizens and their governments. …We have economies that are widely seen as unsustainable, unfair, unstable and deeply unfulfilling. In addition, inter-class mobility is now blocked, even in countries like the U.S. …Economic inequality is now among the two most frequently cited threats to economic stability. …And inequality has grown rapidly in many countries around the world, often fuelled by corruption and excessive greed. …Inequality, even more than poverty, is harmful to everybody in society. Unequal countries have

far more social problems (including crime and corruption), lower trust levels and everybody's well-being is depressed compared to more equal countries. In a similar vein, Nobel Laureate Amartya Sen has argued that those who suffer from inequality (even in wealthy societies) face a diminution in their basic economic and political freedoms—such as their ability to achieve political efficacy.

WEF maintains that moving from a shareholder economy driven by profits for shareholders to a stakeholder economy where business is done in ways that benefit the stakeholders will help to overcome the loss of trust and deep sense of betrayal and unfairness that has grown in societies around the world. The case study in the Afterword gives a concrete example of the deep influence of globalization, economics, and the failure to consider stakeholders on health.

Of Contracts and Covenants

Movement from a shareholder to a stakeholder economy is necessary but not sufficient. WEF proposes that it is also necessary to move from social contract to social covenant:

> We believe that this should be a Covenant not a Contract as values and trust are much more important in a Covenant than in a Contact. A contract is transactional; while a covenant is moral. By definition, this will require the engagement and collaboration of all stakeholders—governments, business, civil society groups, faith groups etc. Such Covenants will vary from country to country, and it is not possible to be prescriptive about either content or process. It is expected though, that certain universal values, such as the dignity of the individual, the primacy of promoting the common good, and the responsibility for stewardship of the planet, will feature in all of them.[76]

The differences between contract and covenant are significant and profound. As WEF notes, contract is transactional (society gives nursing autonomy in exchange for guaranteeing competence). Contract is also minimalist. In the social contract with professions, professions should have the interests of society at heart and not abuse their privilege. While applying them to medicine, William May has identified distinctions between a contract and a covenant:

> Both include an exchange and an agreement between parties. But... contract and covenant are quite different. Contracts are external; covenants are internal to the parties involved. Contracts are signed to be expediently discharged. Covenants have a gratuitous, growing

edge to them that nourishes rather than limits relationships. …There is a donative element in the nourishing of covenant—whether it is the covenant of marriage, friendship, or professional relationship. Tit-for-tat characterizes a commercial transaction, but it does not exhaustively define the vitality of that relationship in which one must serve and draw upon the deeper reserves of another.

The Donative Element of Covenant

In applying covenant to the practice of medicine, May discusses the donative element of covenant. *Donative*, from the Latin *dōnātīvus*, means "gift or donation."[77] There is a gift element, a donative element, in covenant that does not exist in contract:

> This donative element is important not only in the doctor's care of the patient but in other aspects of health care. …The kind of minimalism encouraged by a contractualist understanding of the professional relationship produces a professional too grudging, too calculating, too lacking in spontaneity, too quickly exhausted to go the second mile with his patients along the road of their distress. … Contract medicine not only encourages minimalism, it also provokes a peculiar kind of maximalism, the name for which is "defensive medicine."…Paradoxically, contractualism simultaneously tempts the doctor to do too little and too much for the patient: too little in that one extends oneself only to the limits of what is specified in the contract.[78]

THINKING ABOUT THE DONATIVE ELEMENT…

The concept of the "self-made man" is deeply flawed. It refers to the person who, by dint of her or his own diligence and patient effort, and against all odds, rises above circumstances and makes good, or even better than good—hits the jackpot and becomes wealthy, successful, or famous. However, no one gets there exclusively on her own, and no, you cannot really pull yourself up by your own bootstraps—just try it. Bootstraps don't beat gravity.

My taxes pay for public schools for the children I do not have. Your taxes pay for streets, roads and highways that you will never see. His taxes pay for diversion programs for nurses that he will never use. Her taxes pay for parks that her allergies will not let her visit. This is part of the donative element of society. The self-made person goes to grade school in school buses supported by taxpayers, attends schools supported by taxpayers or philanthropists, on scholarships funded by taxpayers or philanthropists, and that is only the start of indebtedness. There is no such thing as a self-made nurse either. Nursing education and research is supported by federal, state, and philanthropic dollars. But the donative element is much deeper and much more personal than that. People who donate organs and blood, participate in research, and allow student nurses to practice on them are giving very personal gifts in the context of health care. These gifts create a moral milieu of gift–gratitude–indebtedness that is repeated constantly in health care.

We were discussing covenant as social covenant and May has, in these quotes, brought it to the level of individual practitioner. He does read covenant back into a larger societal level, where, in fact, covenant originated:

> The concept of covenant has…further advantages for defining the professional relationship…it is important also for whole institutions—the hospital, the clinic, the professional group—to keep covenant with those who seek their assistance and sanctuary. Thus the concept permits a certain broadening of accountability beyond personal agency to set professional responsibility for this one human good (health) within social limits. The professional covenant concerning health should be situated within a larger set of covenant obligations that both the doctor and patient have toward other institutions and priorities within the society at large. The traditional models for the doctor/patient relationship (parent, friend) tend to establish an exclusivity of relationship that obscures those larger responsibilities.[79]

While there is a body of literature in medicine, and to some degree in nursing, that links covenant to individual practitioners in relationship to patients, the origins of covenant are much larger—and quite ancient.

A History of Covenant

According to Mendenhall and Herion, "covenants in the form of international treaties appeared almost as soon as writing itself began to be used for literary purposes."[80] Examples of covenants can be found from the Early Bronze Age (about 3000 BCE) and the Iron Age (1200–550 BCE), but are best known through the covenants of the Hittite period (1700–1200 BCE). Today covenants are primarily know through the Jewish scriptures of the pre-monarchic period. There were five attributes of these ancient covenants:

> By their very nature, covenants are complex *enactments*. As complex acts they combine: (1) historical events that create relationships, usually (though not necessarily) between unequal partners; (2) customary ways of thinking characteristic of both parties, especially common religious ideas associated with deities; (3) descriptions of norms for future behavior… (4) literary or oral forms in which the agreement is couched; and (5) almost always some ritual act that is regarded as essential to the ratification of the binding promise.[81]

For the purposes of this discussion the second attribute is where we need to turn our attention. Covenants were typically enacted between two parties to create a relationship where one had not existed. By entering into and because of this relationship both parties come to see themselves differently and gain different expectations for themselves and one another. In other words, there is an ontological change in both parties of a covenant, a change in the very nature of being in both parties and who they are, both with one another and in the world. At the personal level, I am changed in the very nature of who I am when I enter into a marriage covenant, as is my spouse. I am changed in the very nature of who I am as a nurse, as is the patient, when we come into relationship with one another for help and healing. This is the antithesis of what nurses were once taught—to stand apart from the patient, and to be the dispassionate, detached nursing caregiver as if we were not touched by the patient.

Nursing's Social Covenant

So I am changed in the nature of who I am by virtue of the covenant relationship; I undergo an ontological change. A part of that change is that the covenant brings me into solidarity with the other person. In covenant relationship, I come to experience, to know (gnosis), intimately, ontologically, the shared human condition. It is also within the context of covenant that I experience the donative element of relationship. Who can forget the willing patient who allows the quivering student to give that very first injection? Or the human participant in nursing research, for whom there is no potential benefit, who willingly donates herself or himself to the research for the benefit of persons she or he will never know—or for the nursing doctoral student struggling to complete dissertation research. There is also the grateful nursing student who survives by having received a federal traineeship funded by the unknown taxpayers, or the researcher who has a federal grant to fund a study, or the school of nursing whose new building was funded by a foundation. The donative element within society abounds, and nursing has been a recipient.

However, we are not focused here on the individual nurse–patient relationship, but rather on the notion of a social covenant. Nursing's history of selfless giving, of supererogation, of exceeding the expectations of the social contract—to the level that it is, as previously noted, regarded as the most trusted profession in the nation—lends itself to understanding nursing's relationship with society as meeting and exceeding the expectations of the social contract that authorizes it, but as going beyond social contract and enacting the nursing–society relationship as social covenant. In a society that disvalues care and care work, nursing has persisted in caring, not with simple competence but with excellence, energy, imagination—and love. In a society that has created health disparities, nursing has come alongside disadvantaged groups and has been an advocate. In a society in which race, class, and gender divisions are both deep and wide, nursing has worked to overcome those divisions both within the profession and in society. In a society that would divide into in-groups and out-groups, separated in part by access to care, nursing has asserted solidarity with all those in need of nursing and has affirmed the consanguinity of human-kind, that is, the kinship of all humanity and the shared human condition. In a society that has allowed self-interest to create harm, nursing has worked dil-igently and altruistically for the common good.[82] Well beyond social contract, nursing engages society as social covenant.

We close with words from the *Code of Ethics for Nurses with Interpretive Statements*, 2015:

> The nursing profession must actively participate in solidarity with the global nursing community and health organizations to represent the collective voice of U.S. nurses around the globe. Professional nursing organizations must actively engage in the political process, particularly in addressing legislative and regulatory concerns that most affect—positively and negatively—the public's health and the profession of nursing. Nurses must promote open and honest com-munication that enables nurses to work in concert, share in scholar-ship, and advance a nursing agenda for health. Global health, as well as the common good, are ideals that can be realized when all nurses unite their efforts and energies. Social justice extends beyond human health and well-being to the health and well-being of the natural world. Human life and health are profoundly affected by the state of the natural world that surrounds us. Consistent with Florence Nightingale's historic concerns for environmental influences on health, and with the metaparadigm of nursing, the profession's advo-cacy for social justice extends to eco-justice. …As nursing seeks to promote and restore health, prevent illness and injury, and alleviate pain and suffering, it does so within the holistic context of healing the world.[83]

Gedankenexperimente: On Civic and Cosmopolite Professionalism, Nursing Education, Power and Value Structures, and Covenant

- Who would you identify as examples of civic or cosmopolite professionalism?

- How should nursing education be changed or restructured to enhance civic and cosmopolite professionalism?

- What would it take for all nurses, not simply nursing students, to experience a cognitive apprenticeship?

- How can nursing educate for episteme, gnosis, and sophia?
- Of the three functions of social ethics, what are your strengths and passions?
- What are ways in which globalization has helped and harmed nursing?
- How can nursing use globalization to further the goal of health for all?
- What power structures most threaten nursing's meaning and value structures?
- In what supererogatory ways does nursing contribute to health?
- What donative elements have benefitted nursing as a profession?
- In what ways does or might nursing operate under a covenant, both nationally and globally?
- What might a written nursing social covenant contain?

ENDNOTES

1   ANA, "Tentative Code," 977.

2   *Oxford English Dictionary Online*, "Cosmopolite," 2015, http://0-www.oed.com. patris.apu.edu/view/Entry/42264?redirectedFrom=cosmopolite&. Access requires login.

3   Sullivan, *Work and Integrity*.

4   Benner et al., *Educating Nurses*.

5   Sullivan and Benner, "Challenges to Professionalism," 79.

6   Benner et al., *Educating Nurses*, 72, 205.

7   Ibid., 166. Italics in original.

8   Ibid., 166, 168.

9   Ibid., 177. Italics in original.

10   ANA, *Code of Ethics for Nurses with Interpretive Statements* (2015), 32.

11   ANA, *Nursing: Scope and Standards of Practice,* (2nd ed.)

12   Vladimir Lossky, *Orthodox Theology* (Crestwood, NY: St. Vladimir's Seminary Press, 1989).

13   Vladimir Lossky, *The Mystical Theology of the Eastern Church* (Crestwood, NY: St. Vladimir's Seminary Press, 1976). See also: Georges Florovsky, *The Ways of Russian Theology*, trans. Robert Nichols, vols. 1 and 2 (Belmont, MA: Norland, 1979); and Sergius Bulgakov, *The Orthodox Church* (Crestwood, NY: St. Vladimir's Seminary Press, 1988).

14   Marsha Fowler, "Spirituality, Faith and Nursing Practice," in *Conference Papers: New Nurses for a New Russia* (Golitsino, RU: 1994), originally published in Russian. See also: Fowler, "Social Ethics and the Role of Professional Associations," in *Conference Papers: New Nurses for a New Russia* (Golitsino, RU: 1994), originally published in Russian.; Fowler, *Central Themes in Russian Orthodox Christianity and the Concept of Health* (Moscow: Ministry of Health, 1994), originally published in Russian; and Fowler, *Spirituality, Faith and Health* (Moscow: Ministry of Health, 1994), originally published in Russian.

15   Benner et al., *Educating Nurses*, 210.

16   Fowler, *Guide to the Code of Ethics*.

17   Gibson Winter, *Elements for a Social Ethics* (New York: Macmillan, 1966), 215.

18   Fowler, *Guide to the Code of Ethics*, 152.

19   This section on social ethics modified from: Fowler, *Guide to the Code of Ethics*, 152–55.

20   Fowler, "Social Ethics and Nursing," 24–30. See also: Fowler, "Professional Associations, Ethics and Society," *Oncology Nursing Forum* 20, no. 10 (November/ December 1993): 13–19.

21   Evelyn Barbee, "Racism in U.S. Nursing," *Medical Anthropology Quarterly* 7, no. 4 (December 1993): 346–62. See also: Pamela Brink, "Cultural Diversity in Nursing: How Much Can We Tolerate?" in *Current Issues in Nursing*, ed. Joanne C. McCloskey and Helen K.Grace, 3rd ed. (St. Louis, MO: C. V. Mosby, 1990), 521– 27; and Mary E. Carnagie, *The Path We Tread: Blacks in Nursing 1854-1990*, 2nd ed. (New York: National League for Nursing, 1991).

22   Pam Smith and Maureen Macintosh, "Profession, Market and Class: Nurse Migration and the Remaking of Division and Disadvantage," *Journal of Clinical Nursing*, 2007: 2213–20. See also: Kimberly A. Van Herk, Dawn Smith, and Caroline Andrew, "Examining Our Privileges and Oppressions: Incorporating Intersectionality Paradigm into Nursing," *Nursing Inquiry* 18, no. 1 (March 2011): 29–39; Bukola Salami and Sioban Nelson, "The Downward Occupational Mobility of Internationally Educated Nurses to Domestic Workers," *Nursing Inquiry* 21, no. 2 (June 2014): 153–61; Carol Helmstadter, "Shifting Boundaries; Religion, Medicine, Nursing and Domestic Service in Mid-Nineteenth-Century Britain," *Nursing Inquiry* 16, no. 2 (June 2009): 133–43; Williams, Muller, Kilanski, "Gendered Organizations," 549–73; and Nono Glazer, "'Between a Rock and a Hard Place': Women's Professional Organizations in Nursing and Class, Racial, and Ethnic Inequalities," *Gender and Society* 5, no. 3 (Sept 1991): 351–72.

23   C. Perelman and L. Olbrechts-Tyteca, *The New Rhetoric: A Treatise on Argumentation*, trans. John Wilkinson and Purcell Weaver (Notre Dame, IN: University of Notre Dame Press, 1969), 51.

24   Ibid.

25 ANA, "Suggested Code," 599.

26 ANA, *Code of Ethics for Nurses* (2015), 31.

27 World Health Organization, *Closing the Gap: Policy into Practice on Social Determinants of Health* (Geneva: WHO, 2011), 2; World Health Organization, *Meeting Report of the World Conference on Social Determinants of Health* in Rio de Janeiro, Brazil, October 19–21, 2011 (Geneva: WHO, 2012), ix.

28 M. Horkheimer, *Critical Theory* (New York: Seabury Press, 1982), 244.

29 Committee on the Robert Wood Johnson Foundation Initiative on the Future of Nursing, *Future of Nursing*, 8.

30 "Apply Now for Government Affairs Internship," American Association of Colleges of Nursing, http://www.aacn.nche.edu/government-affairs/internship. See also: "IOM/AAN/ANA/ANF Distinguished Nurse Scholar in Residence," Institute of Medicine, http://www.iom.edu/Activities/Education/NurseScholar.aspx; "The Fellowship," Nursing and Health Policy Collaborative, http://nursinghealthpolicy.org/the-fellowship/; "Robert Wood Johnson Foundation Health Policy Fellows," Robert Wood Johnson Foundation, http://www.rwjfleaders.org/programs/robert-wood-johnson-foundation-health-policy-fellow; and Rachel Watman, "New Nurse Fellowship Will Help Prepare Gero-Focused Policy Leaders," The John A. Hartford Foundation, updated February 19, 2013, http://www.jhartfound.org/blog/new-nurse-fellowship-will-help-prepare-gero-focused-policy-leaders/.

31 Sullivan, *Work and Integrity*, 208.

32 John Fien, "Globalisation," written for United Nations Education, Scientific and Cultural Organization (UNESCO), http://www.unesco.org/education/tlsf/mods/theme_c/mod18.html.

33 Sobhi Tawil, "Education for 'Global Citizenship': A Framework for Discussion," *UNESCO Education Research and Foresight Working Papers*, no. 7 (August 2013): 6, http://unesdoc.unesco.org/images/0022/002237/223784e.pdf.

34 Ibid., 2. See also: R. Falk, "The Making of Global Citizenship," in *The Condition of Citizenship*, ed. B. Van Steenbergen (London: Sage Publications, 1994); and M. E. Keck and K. Sikkink, *Activists Beyond Borders* (Ithaca, NY: Cornell University Press, 1998).

35 K. A. Appiah, "Education for Global Citizenship: A Framework for Discussion," in *Yearbook of the National Society for the Study of Education*, ed. D. Coulter, G. Fenstermacher, and J. R. Wiens, vol. 1 (New York: The National Society for the Study of Education/Teachers' College Columbia, 2008).

36 Appiah, "Education for Global Citizenship," 2. Italics in original.

37 Ibid. Error in original.

38 Ibid., 5.

39 Ibid., 6.

40 UNESCO, *Global Citizenship Education: Preparing Learners for the Challenges of the Twenty-First Century* (Paris: UNESCO, 2014), http://unesdoc.unesco.org/images/0022/002277/227729E.pdf.

41 Anita Finkelman and Carole Kenner, *Teaching IOM: Implications of the Institute of Medicine Reports for Nursing Education*, 3rd ed. (Silver Spring, MD: American Nurses Association, 2012).

42 International Conference on Primary Health Care, *Declaration of Alma-Ata* (Alma-Ata, USSR, September 1978).

43 "Background," U.N. Millennium Development Goals, http://www.un.org/millenniumgoals/bkgd.shtml.

44 Anita Hunter et al., "Global Health Diplomacy: An Integrative Review of the Literature and Implications for Nursing," *Nursing Outlook* 61, no. 2 (2013): 85. See also: J. B. Koplan et al., "Towards a common definition of global health," *Lancet* 373 (2009): 1993–1995.

45 Jean-Jacques Rousseau, *A Discourse on the Origin of Inequality and A Discourse on Political Economy*, trans. G. D. H. Cole, 3rd ed. (New York: Digireads, 2005), 74.

46 Ibid., 77.

47 Martha Nussbaum, *Creating Capabilities: The Human Development Approach* (Cambridge, MA: Harvard/Belknap, 2011). See also: Nussbaum, *Frontiers of Justice: Disability, Nationality, Species Membership* (Cambridge, MA: Harvard/Belknap, 2006); and Nussbaum, *Women and Human Development: The Capabilities Approach*, The Seeley Lectures (Cambridge, UK: Cambridge University Press, 2001).

48 Nussbaum, *Creating Capabilities*, 85.

49 Ibid.

50 Ibid., 87.

51 Ibid., 86.

52 Nussbaum, *Creating Capabilities*, 186.

53 Tronto, *Moral Boundaries*, 178.

54 Ibid., 35–36, 50–58.

55 Ibid., 161.

56 Ibid., 169.

57 Ibid., 162–67.

58 Ibid., 77.

59 Ibid., 87.

60 Charles Raith II, "Calvin's Critique of Merit, and why Aquinas (Mostly) Agrees," *Pro Ecclesia* 20, no. 2 (2011): 135–66.

61 Robert Eisen, "*Lifnim Mi-shurat Ha-din* in Maimonides *Mishneh Torah*," *Jewish Quarterly Review* 89, no. 3/4 (January/April 1999): 291–317.

62 J. Urmson, "Saints and Heroes," in *Essays in Moral Philosophy*, ed. A. I. Melden (Seattle: University of Washington Press, 1958).

63 "Clara Louise Maass," American Association for the History of Nursing, http://www.aahn.org/gravesites/maass.html.

64 Clara D. Noyes, "American Nurses' Memorial, Bordeaux, France," *American Journal of Nursing* 24, no. 3 (March 1924): 192.

65 Jacobellis v. Ohio, 378 U.S. 184 (1964), https://supreme.justia.com/cases/federal/us/378/184/case.html.

66 Eric Beerbohm and Ryan Davis, "The Common Good: A Buck-Passing Account," Manuscript/working paper, (Boston: Harvard University Press, forthcoming), 18, http://www.gov.harvard.edu/files/ebrdcommongoodbuckpass.pdf.

67 Pope Paul VI, *Pastoral Constitution on the Church in the Modern World:* Gaudium et Spes (December 7, 1965), Section 26. http://www.vatican.va/archive/ hist_councils/ii_vatican_council/documents/vat-ii_cons_19651207_gaudium-et-spes_en.html. Italics added.

68 The Catholic Bishops' Conference of England and Wales, *The Common Good and the Catholic Church's Social Teaching* (1996), 15, http://www.catholicsocialteaching. org.uk/wp-content/uploads/2010/10/THE-COMMON-GOOD-AND-THE-CATHOLIC-CHURCH_1996.pdf.

69 Ibid., 19.

70 Henri-Claude de Bettignies and Françoise Lépineux, *Business, Globalization and the Common Good* (Oxford, UK: Peter Lang, 2009), 38.

71 Ibid.

72 "Our Members," World Economic Forum, http://www.weforum.org/our-members.

73 Ibid.

74 "A New Social Contract," WEF Global Agenda Council on Values (Davos-Klosters, Switzerland: January 23–27 2013), http://www3.weforum.org/docs/WEF_GAC_Values_2013.pdf.

75 Ibid., 4.

76 Ibid., 5.

77 *Oxford English Dictionary Online*, "Donative," http://0-www.oed.com.patris.apu. edu/view/Entry/56745?redirectedFrom=donative#eid. Access requires login.

78 William F. May, "Code, Covenant, Contract and Philanthropy," *Hastings Center Report* 5, no. 6 (December 1975): 34–35.

79 Ibid., 36.

80 George E. Mendenhall, and Gary A. Herion, "Covenant," in *The Anchor Yale Bible Dictionary*, vol. 1, *A—C*, ed. David Noel Freedman (New Haven, CT: Yale University Press, 1992), 1180.

81 Ibid.

82 Sylvia Walby, "Analyzing Social Inequality in the Twenty-First Century: Globalization and Modernity Restructure Inequality," *Contemporary Sociology* 29, no. 6 (November 2000): 813–18. See also: Rachel E. Dwyer, "The Care Economy? Gender, Economic Restructuring, and Job Polarization in the US Labor Market," *American Sociological Review* 78, no. 3 (November 2013): 390–416; Philip N. Cohen and Matt L. Huffman, "Individuals, Jobs, and Labor Markets: The Devaluation of Women's Work," *American Sociological Review* 68, no. 3 (June 2003): 443–63; Marshall, "Recent History of Professionalism," 325–40; Chang Hwan Kim, "The Rise of Intra-Occupational Wage Inequality in the United States, 1983 to 2002," *American Sociological Review* 73, no. 1 (February 2008): 129–57; and Parsons, "Professions and Social Structure," 457–67.

83 ANA, *Code of Ethics for Nurses* (2015), 36–37.

Afterword
Why All This Matters

The content of the preceding four chapters does not have immediate or direct connection to everyday clinical practice, so it raises the question "Why does this matter?" It matters in several ways.

The concepts developed in this book provide a framework for understanding nursing's social contract and the mutual expectations of that contract. However, for those who have an insatiable curiosity, understanding alone is not adequate. As the concepts herein provide a framework for understanding the social contract, they also provide a framework for its analysis and critique informed by a range of intersectional and critical theories. These theories help identify where change is needed and, in part, what it might take to bring about change. Nursing education that is formative in the values of the profession and in ethical comportment, is also formative of a disposition to action—action that implements nursing values. Understanding is essential but not sufficient. Nurses' disposition to action is first built upon understanding. It then moves to assessment, data collection, planning, action, and evaluation: the nursing process, our profession's own approach to critical thinking.

Many of the persistent issues in health, both national and global, endure because their origins do not reside in bacteria: the causes are social. As such, they are complex, political, cultural, and refractory to change. That does not mean that nursing efforts should not be applied to seek their amelioration or resolution. It does mean that nurses must understand the complexity and parameters of global issues and then work collectively, in concert and in collaboration, on many fronts. There is more than enough work to go around, which means that individual nurses can contribute at any level, and in any number of ways, in accord with their interests, passions, knowledge, and skills. Cosmopolite professionalism requires both individual and collective global engagement to address socially constructed health problems. We turn now to one example, that of the feminization of HIV/AIDS. This case issue is chosen because it touches upon a number of contributory factors, some of which may be unexpected.

Global Example: The Feminization of HIV/AIDS

Since the late 1990s, there has been and continues to be more than ample international documentation of the feminization of HIV/AIDs globally, but particularly in sub-Saharan Africa. Klot and Nguyen write that

> the HIV and AIDS pandemic both fuels and is fuelled by inequalities across gender, race, ethnicity and class. Its effects vary across different settings and regions of the world and are also shaped by armed conflicts, natural disasters, environmental degradation, state incapacities, famine and poverty. Its refractory impacts on women and girls—and humanity writ large—are nothing short of catastrophic.

> The third decade of the pandemic is characterized by sub-epidemics that are now coursing through many parts of the globe and among groups previously considered to be unaffected. Growing and disproportionate impacts are now being seen among young women and girls, particularly in sub-Saharan Africa, where young women between 15 and 24 years old are at least three times more likely to be HIV-positive than young men. Nearly half the 30.8 million people living with HIV worldwide are women between the ages of 15 and 49. Between the ages of 15 and 24, gender disparities are even more extreme, with women 1.5 times more likely to be living with HIV than young men (UNAIDS, 2008).[1]

This trend continues to grow. However, the causes of this disproportionate impact are not biological; they are a consequence of a cataclysm of social causes. Again, Klot and Nguyen note the following:

> In different settings and epidemics, mainstream approaches ignore the most basic driver of the pandemic: the *unequal power relations* between women and men, girls and boys. The power structures that determine women's and men's different abilities to protect themselves from infection; to access quality prevention, treatment and care; and to cope with the consequences of the pandemic are poorly understood. These structures have also received scant policy attention, making it difficult for practitioners and policy-makers to understand the specificities of each epidemic and to identify what should be done differently to address them.[2]

As part of the power structures of this issue, some of the cultural practices that elevate the risk of girls and women to HIV/AIDS include: underage female marriage, female genital mutilation (FGM) or cutting, wife inheritance, widow cleansing, infant/virgin rape, polygamy when the husband is HIV positive, prohibitions against male circumcision, denial of reproductive education to females, rape as an instrument of war, and more.[3]

Power structures have overwhelmed meaning and value structures (and we shall return shortly to contributory aspects of the power structures that disadvantage females). Klot, Nugyen, and colleagues implicate gender and violence, specifically sexual violence, as well as race, class, and ethnicity in the catastrophic elevation of risk for women and girls. Any single aspect of these linkages is fertile ground for nursing research and action and makes clear the importance of intersectionality in such research. Clearly, these linkages are not unique to HIV/AIDS; they have implications for women and women's health in many spheres. Klot and Nguyen's work *The Fourth Wave: Violence, Gender, Culture and HIV in the 21st Century* has methodological, epistemological, and critical social theory explorations that have a wide range of applicability outside of HIV/AIDS.

Structural Adjustment Policies and the Social Safety Net: Health Consequences

Let's look at one—only one of many—less obvious element of power structures that has a profound influence on women's health in less-developed countries, specifically poorer, or debtor, countries. We noted in Chapter 4 that globalization is fundamentally economic in nature. UNESCO identifies the first precept of globalization as "the acceptance of a set of economic rules for the entire world designed to maximise profits and productivity by universalising markets and production, and to obtain the support of the state with a view to making the national economy more productive and competitive."[4] As we reflect on pandemics, and even the devastation of large-scale natural disasters, we do not immediately link issues of trade, markets, and production to health. However, they are intimately intertwined.

When developing countries need to borrow from the World Bank[5] (WB) or the International Monetary Fund[6] (IMF) they qualify for loans by becoming subject to a set of *structural adjustment policies* (SAPs) within the Structural Adjustment Programmes. These policies are

> economic policies for developing countries that have been promoted
> by the World Bank and International Monetary Fund (IMF) since
> the early 1980s by the provision of loans [to low-income nations]
> conditional on the adoption of…policies…designed to encourage
> the structural adjustment of an economy by, for example, removing
> "excess" government controls and promoting market competition. …
> One important criticism of SAPs, which emerged shortly after they

were first adopted and has continued since, concerns their impact on the social sector. In health, SAPs affect both the supply of health services (by insisting on cuts in health spending) and the demand for health services (by reducing household income, thus leaving people with less money for health). Studies have shown that SAPs have slowed down improvements in, or worsened, the health status of people in countries implementing them. The results reported include worse nutritional status of children, increased incidence of infectious diseases, and higher infant and maternal mortality rates.[7]

The World Bank itself acknowledges the devastating effects of the SAPs upon health. In its 2002 report, it notes that SAPs

> have had a profound effect on all aspects of political, social and economic life in developing and transition countries. That impact has been felt quite deeply in the social sector. Civil-society organizations, often joined by United Nations agencies like UNICEF, have been particularly critical of the impact on the poor of large budgetary cuts in such areas as health care and education carried out under adjustment programs over the past two decades. The social sector is also one of the areas in which the World Bank has found itself vulnerable to the charge that its policies are disproportionately hurting the poor.[8]

In the SAP scales, economics is weighted more heavily than the social safety net. How does this weigh out in terms of HIV/AIDS? At the risk of being reductive, here is a concise picture of the cycle. Often structural adjustment policies require borrowing countries to reduce expenditures supporting the social safety net, including expenditures on health, sanitation, education, water delivery systems and purification, social welfare, and more. They also require the removal of subsidies and price controls designed to control the prices of, for example, food and milk. In addition, these SAPs require trade adjustments, including the reduction of trade barriers, enhancements in the rights of foreign investors (increased foreign direct investment), market deregulation, and privatization or divestiture of state enterprises, the devaluation of the nation's currency, cutting wages, and focusing on economic output (export production) and resource extraction. Devaluing currency while removing price controls results in an immediate increase in prices (on the order of three to four times higher), the consequence of which is increased poverty within the nation, giving rise, in some cases, to riots.[9] Because of the negative consequences and reputation of the SAPs, there has been some revision:

SAPs have now largely been replaced by the Poverty Reduction Strategy Paper (PRSP) process. Also, World Bank operational guidelines now require analysis of the impact of adjustment programmes on the poor and, in many countries, compensatory measures have been introduced. Critics argue that this is a "social safety net approach" in which social services are not regarded as a part of the normal primary functions of the modern state, but rather as institutions that respond to market failure.[10]

However, the Structural Adjustment Participatory Review International Network (SAPRIN) four-year study, a multinational investigation of the SAPs, shows continuing effects upon social safety nets, including on poverty, hunger, health, employment, and more.

SAPs and HIV/AIDS Among Women

In addition to the impacts of SAPs on employment, health, education, hunger, and poverty, cuts in social expenditures have profoundly gendered effects across all of these domains. The burden of providing for health, sanitation, food preparation, and welfare culturally falls disproportionately on women, often women already living in abject poverty. As jobs move into urban areas, rural men out-migrate to cities for manufacturing jobs, leaving women and children behind to fend for themselves in the rural areas (referred to as the *feminization of agriculture*).[11] Sex workers, at times provided by employers, cluster near factories. Some of these men begin second families near the factory. Men who become HIV infected transmit this to their spouse or spouses when they visit their families in the rural areas. Already suffering from typically unequal sexual power relations that increase their risk, these women often cannot refuse unprotected sex with a spouse. The women have also borne an increased vulnerability through their hardscrabble economic status, which renders them unable to seek medical treatment or health/reproductive care, both because of poverty and cultural influences. This has likewise increased the vulnerability of their children to disease, while the poverty also assures that their children will suffer a lack of education and food insecurity.[12]

In response to the adverse consequences of the SAPs for health, well-being, hunger, poverty, education, employment, and more, George notes that

> debt is an efficient tool. It ensures access to other peoples' raw materials and infrastructure on the cheapest possible terms. Dozens of countries must compete for shrinking export markets and can export only a limited range of products because of Northern protectionism and their lack of cash to invest in diversification. Market saturation ensues, reducing exporters' income to a bare minimum while the

North enjoys huge savings. The IMF cannot seem to understand that investing in…[a] healthy, well-fed, literate population…is the most intelligent economic choice a country can make.[13]

Here we have the clash of power structures with meaning and value structures, and power structures have won out. There are multiple points at which the vicissitudes of SAPs in relation to health can be addressed by nursing, but one approach is that of health diplomacy as discussed in Chapter 4.[14] If nursing wishes to make a difference in global health, it needs to identify which fronts and with whom it will mount an attack to bring about change(s). The questions below are intended to provoke thinking about nursing, its global engagement, and global health.

Gedankenexperimente: On the Feminization of HIV/AIDS, Global Health, and Nursing's Cosmopolite Professionalism

Using this case issue as an example, you are invited to set aside any concerns for financing or other barriers and to dream big.

- What curricular changes need to be made to equip nurses to assess global health issues and plan for intervention?

- What educational preparation (content) would be necessary to create a cadre of nurses equipped to engage in health diplomacy?

- What would a cognitive apprenticeship include in order to create a formative education for involvement with global health?

- With whom, specifically, could nursing organizations partner for involvement?

- What kinds of nursing research are needed to address the feminization of HIV/AIDS?

- What are ways in which an individual nurse might contribute to nursing's collective efforts to halt the feminization of HIV/AIDS, from a local, regional, state, national, or international base?

- What might be examples of the smallest manageable unit for effective global engagement for individual nurses that any nurse might do?

- What are examples of outsized nursing contributions to global health?

- Who are the nursing leaders and emerging leaders in global health?

- How would you communicate to a nurse working in your local community hospital that she or he can contribute to resolving the feminization of HIV/AIDS (or any global health issue)?

ENDNOTES

1   Jennifer Klot and Vinh-Kim Nguyen, ed., *The Fourth Wave: Violence, Gender, Culture & HIV in the 21st Century* (Paris: UNESCO, 2011), 15.

2   Ibid., 11. Italics added.

3   Advisory Committee on Social Witness Policy, Presbyterian Church (USA), *Becoming an HIV and AIDS Competent Church: Prophetic Witness and Compassionate Action* (Louisville, KY: Presbyterian Church, 2010), 18–20. *Note:* Author was a member and lead writer of the team that created this document. See also: Stephen Buckley, "Wife Inheritance Spurs AIDS Rise in Kenya," *Washington Post Foreign Service*, Saturday, November 8, 1997, http://www. washingtonpost.com/wp-srv/inatl/longterm/africanlives/kenya/kenya_aids.htm; J. P. Owino, "Wife Inheritance and 'Chira' Cultural Impediments in HIV and AIDS Control, Prevention and Management: A Case Study of Luo Community in Kenya," *International Conference on AIDS* 12 (1998): 474; Uche U. Ewelukwa, "Post-Colonialism, Gender, Customary Injustice: Widows in African Societies," *Human Rights Quarterly* 24, no. 2 (May, 2002): 424–86; B. L. Meel, "The Myth of Child Rape as a Cure for HIV/AIDS in Transkei: A Case Report," *Medicine, Science and the Law* 43 (2003): 85–88; N.E. Groce and R. Trasi, "Rape of Individuals with Disability: AIDS and the Folk Belief of Virgin Cleansing," *Lancet* 363 (2004): 1663–64; M. K. Nsubuga et al., "The Dilemmas of Cultural Reforms in the Era of HIV/AIDS: The Case of Polygamy in the Muslim Community in Uganda," *International Conference on AIDS* 12 (1998): 231; S. Seck, "Migration, Polygamy and HIV-SIDA (The Experience of Senegalese Women Infected with HIV/SIDA)," *International Conference on AIDS* 13 (July 19–14 2000); and WHO/UNAIDS Technical Consultation Male Circumcision and HIV Prevention, "New Data on Male Circumcision and HIV Prevention: Policy and Programme Implications" (Montreau, Switzerland: WHO, March 2007), http://libdoc.who.int/publications/2007/9789241595988_eng.pdf.

4   John Fien, "Globalisation," written for United Nations Education, Scientific and Cultural Organization (UNESCO), http://www.unesco.org/education/tlsf/mods/theme_c/mod18.html.

5   "What We Do," World Bank, http://www.worldbank.org/en/about/what-we-do.

6   "The IMF at a Glance," International Monetary Fund, http://www.imf.org/external/np/exr/facts/glance.htm.

7   "Structural Adjustment Programmes (SAPs)," World Health Organization, http://www.who.int/trade/glossary/story084/en/.

8   Structural Adjustment Participatory Review International Network (SAPRIN), *The Policy Roots of Economic Crisis and Poverty* (Washington, DC: SAPRIN, April 2002), 147.

9   Susan George, *A Fate Worse Than Debt* (New York: Grove Weidenfeld, 1990).

10 "Adjustment with a Human Face," World Health Organization, http://www.who.int/trade/glossary/story003/en/.

11 Ann Whitehead, "The Gendered Impacts of Liberalization Policies on African Agricultural Economies and Rural Livelihoods," in *Gender Equality: Striving for Justice in an Unequal World*, a UN Research Institute for Social Development report (New York: Routledge, 2009), 37–62, http://www.unrisd.org/80256B3C005B CCF9%2F(httpAuxPages)%2FD5B4FE38226FEA6FC125706E00345465% 2F$file%2Fwhitehea.pdf; See also: Carmen Deere, "The Feminization of Agriculture? The Impact of Economic Restructuring in Rural Latin America," In Razavi, *Gendered Impacts of Liberalization*, 99–127.

12 Modified from: Advisory Committee on Social Witness Policy, Presbyterian Church, *Prophetic Witness and Compassionate Action*, 24–26. Though a somewhat polemic work, see also: Rick Rowden, *The Deadly Ideas of Neoliberalism: How the IMF has Undermined Public Health and the Fight Against AIDS* (London: Zed Books, 2009).

13 George, *Fate Worse Than Debt*, 143, 187, 235.

14 Anita Hunter et al., "Global Health Diplomacy," 85.

References and Bibliography

All URLs were current as of May 29, 2015.

Ahmad, Khurshid. "The Challenge of Global Capitalism: An Islamic Perspective." In Dunning, *Making Globalization Good*, 181–209. Oxford, UK: Oxford University Press, 2003.

Allen, Phillip M. Review of *Medicine and the Reign of Technology* by Stanley Joel Reiser. *Medical Anthropology Newsletter* 10, no. 3 (1979): 18.

American Medical Association. *Code of Medical Ethics of the American Medical Association.* Chicago, IL: American Medical Association, 1847.

American Nurses Association. "A Code for Professional Nurses." *American Journal of Nursing* 60, no. 9 (1960): 1227.

———. *Code of Ethics for Nurses with Interpretive Statements.* Silver Spring, MD: American Nurses Association, 2015.

———. "First Position on Education for Nursing." *American Journal of Nursing* 65, no. 12 (1965): 106–11.

———. *Nursing: Scope and Standards of Practice.* 2nd ed. Silver Spring, MD: Nursesbooks.org, 2010.

———. *Nursing's Social Policy Statement: The Essence of the Profession.* Silver Spring, MD: Nursesbooks.org, 2010 in *Nursing: Scope and Standards of Practice.* 3rd ed. Silver Spring, MD: American Nurses Association, 2015.

———. "A Suggested Code." *American Journal of Nursing* 26, no. 8 (1926): 599–600.

———. "A Tentative Code." *American Journal of Nursing* 40, no. 9 (1940): 977–80.

Annas, George J., and Michael A. Grodin. *The Nazi Doctors and the Nuremberg Code.* New York: Oxford University Press, 1992.

Antony, Louise M., and Charlotte Witt, ed. *A Mind of One's Own: Feminist Essays on Reason and Objectivity.* 2nd ed. Boulder, CO: Westview Press, 1993.

Arnot, M. "A Global Conscience Collective? Incorporating Gender Injustices into Global Citizenship Education." *Education, Citizenship and Social Justice* 4, no. 2 (2009): 117–32.

Arruñada, Benito. "Protestants and Catholics: Similar Work Ethic, Different Social Ethic." *Rochester: Social Science Research Network Electronic Journal* (2010).

Austin, Wendy. "Nursing Ethics in an Era of Globalization." *Advances in Nursing Science* 24, no. 2 (2001): 1–18.

Baier, Annette. *Moral Prejudices: Essays on Ethics.* Cambridge, MA: Harvard University Press, 1994.

Baier, Annette C. *Moral Prejudices: Essays on Ethics.* 2nd ed. Cambridge, MA: Harvard University Press, 1995.

Bailey, Michael, and Des Freedman, ed. *The Assault on Universities: A Manifesto for Resistance.* New York: Palgrave Macmillan, 2011.

Baldwin, Dee, and Tommie Nelms. "Difficult Dialogues: Impact on Nursing Education Curricula." *Journal of Professional Nursing* 9, no. 6 (1993): 343–46.

Barbee, Evelyn L. "Racism in U. S. Nursing." *Medical Anthropology Quarterly* 7, no. 4 (December 1993):346–62.

Baron, Marcia. "Kantian Ethics and Supererogation." *Journal of Philosophy* 84, no. 5 (May 1987): 237–62.

Bedke, Matt. "Passing the Deontic Buck." *Oxford Studies in Metaethics* 6 (2011): 128–52.

Beecher, Henry K. "Ethics and Clinical Research." *New England Journal of Medicine* 274, no. 24 (June 16, 1966): 1354–60. Also reproduced with a short, insightful article: Harkness, Jon, Susan E. Lederer, and Daniel Wikler. *Bulletin of the World Health Organization* 79, no. 4 (2001): 365–372.

Bellah, Robert N., Richard Madsen, William M. Sullivan, Ann Swidler, and Steven Tipton. *Habits of the Heart: Individualism and Commitment in American Life*. New York: Harper Perennial, 1986.

———. *The Good Society*. New York: Vintage Books/Random House, 1992.

Benatar, Solomon R., Abdallah S. Daar, and Peter A. Singer. "Global Health Ethics: The Rationale for Mutual Caring." *International Affairs (Royal Institute of International Affairs)* 79, no. 1 (January 2003): 107–38.

Benedict, Susan, Arthur Caplan, and Traute Lafrenz Page. "Duty and 'Euthanasia': The Nurses of Meseritz-Obrawalde." *Nursing Ethics* 14, no. 6 (2007): 781–94.

Benjamin, Martin, Robert M. Veatch, and Sara T. Fry. "Nursing Ethics: An Emerging Integrity." *Hastings Center Report* 18, no. 2 (April–May 1988): 38–39.

Benner, Patricia. "The Role of Experience, Narrative, and Community in Skilled Ethical Comportment." *Advances in Nursing Science* 14, no. 2 (1991): 1–21.

Benner, Patricia, Victoria Leonard, Lisa Day, Molly Sutphen, and Lee S. Shulman. *Educating Nurses: A Call for Radical Transformation*. Jossey-Bass/Carnegie Foundation for the Advancement of Teaching Series. San Francisco: John Wiley & Sons, 2009.

Berger, Peter L., Brigitte Berger, and Hansfried Kellner. *The Homeless Mind: Modernization and Consciousness*. New York: Random House, 1973.

Birsch, Douglas, and John H. Fielder. 1994. *Ford Pinto Case: Study in Applied Ethics, Business and Technology*. Albany: State University of New York Press.

Bixler, Genevieve K., and Roy W. Bixler. "The Professional Status of Nursing." *American Journal of Nursing* 45, no. 9 (1945): 730–35.

———. "The Professional Status of Nursing." *American Journal of Nursing* 59, no. 8 (August 1959): 1142–46.

Blair-Loy, Mary. Review of *People at Work: Life, Power, and Social Inclusion in the New Economy* by Marjorie L. DeVault. *Contemporary Sociology* 38, no. 2 (March 2009): 200–1.

Blumenstyk, Goldie. "Knowledge Is a 'Form of Venture Capital' for a Top Columbia Administrator." *Chronicle of Higher Education,* February 9. http://m.chronicle.com/article/Knowledge-Is-a-Form-of/17565.

Bochenek, Michael P. Review of *Changing Contours of Work: Jobs and Opportunities in the New Economy* by Stephen Sweet and Peter Meiksins. *Teaching Sociology* 36, no. 4 (2008): 396–98. Accessed May 6, 2015. http://www.jstor.org/stable/20491272.

Boucher, David, and Paul Kelly. "The Social Contract and Its Critics: An Overview." In Kelly and Boucher, *The Social Contract from Hobbes to Rawls*, 1–34. New York: Taylor & Francis, 1994.

Bouma, Hessel. "Ethical Considerations in Human Cloning." *Surgery* 125, no. 5 (1999): 468–70.

Boxer, Bruce Alan. "Can Society Take God's Place? A Reflection on Nursing's Social Policy." *Nursing Forum* 43, no. 4 (2008): 247–49.

Boyte, Harry, and Eric Fretz. "Civic Professionalism." *Journal of Higher Education Outreach and Engagement* 1, no. 2 (2010): 69.

Brink, Pamela. "Cultural Diversity in Nursing: How Much Can We Tolerate?" In *Current Issues in Nursing*, edited by Joanne C. McClosky and Helen K. Grace. 3rd ed. 1990.

Brint, Steven G. *In an Age of Experts: Changing Role of Professionals in Politics and Public Life.* Princeton, NJ: Princeton University Press, 1994.

Brody, Howard, and David Doukas. "Professionalism: A Framework to Guide Medical Education." *Medical Education* 48, no. 10 (2014): 980–87.

Buckley, Stephen. "Wife Inheritance Spurs AIDS Rise in Kenya." *Washington Post Foreign Service*, November 8,1997. http://www.washingtonpost.com/wp-srv/inatl/longterm/africanlives/kenya/kenya_aids.htm.

Bulgakov, Sergei Nikolaevich. *The Orthodox Church.* Translated by Lydia W. Kesich and Thomas Hopko. Crestwood, NY: St Vladimir's Seminary Press, 1988.

Byrne, J. "Why I Am Not a Buddhist Feminist: A Critical Examination of 'Buddhist Feminism.'" *Feminist Theology* 21, no. 2 (2012): 180–94.

Cabrera, Luis. *The Practice of Global Citizenship.* Cambridge, UK: Cambridge University Press, 2010.

Cahill, Lisa Sowle. "The Catholic Tradition: Religion, Morality, and the Common Good." *Journal of Law and Religion* 5, no. 1 (1987): 75–94.

Caldwell, Victor F., and Kimberle Williams Crenshaw. "Critical Race Theory: The Key Writings That Formed the Movement." *Columbia Law Review* 96, no. 5 (1996): 1363–74.

Calvin, Jean. *Calvin: Institutes of Christian Religion.* vol 1. Edited by Ford Lewis Battles. Philadelphia: Westminster John Knox Press., 1960.

Caplow, Theodore. *The Sociology of Work.* Minneapolis: University of Minnesota Press, 1954.

Carnegie, Mary Elizabeth. *The Path We Tread: Blacks in Nursing Worldwide 1854-1994.* Sudbury, MA: Jones and Bartlett Publishers, 1999.

Carr, Earl. "Evolution of Nursing." *Journal of the Michigan State Medical Society* 17, no. 5 (May 1915): 186–188.

Carr-Saunders, Alexander M., and Paul A. Wilson. *The Professions.* Oxford, UK: Oxford/Clarendon Press, 1933.

The Catholic Bishops' Conference of England and Wales. "The Common Good and the Catholic Church's Social Teaching." A statement presented by the Catholic Bishops' Conference of England and Wales, 1996. http://www.catholicsocialteaching.org.uk/wp-content/uploads/2010/10/THE-COMMON-GOOD-AND-THE-CATHOLIC-CHURCH_1996.pdf.

Ceh, S., and L. Brian. Review of *Creating the New Economy: The Entrepreneur and the US Resurgence* by R. D. Norton. *Economic Geography* 79, no. 2 (April 2003): 218–19.

Chaska, Norma L., ed. *The Nursing Profession: Turning Points.* St. Louis, MO: C.V. Mosby, 1990.

Cheetham, Graham, and Geoff Chivers. *Professions, Competence and Informal Learning: The Nature of Professions and the Role of Informal Learning in Acquiring Professional Competence.* Cheltenham, UK: Edward Elgar Publishing, 2005.

Cho, Sumi, Kimberlé Williams Crenshaw, and Leslie McCall. "Toward a Field of Intersectionality Studies: Theory, Applications, and Praxis." *Signs* 38, no. 4 (2013): 785–810.

Coffey, Sue. "The Nurse-Patient Relationship in Cancer Care as a Shared Covenant." *Advances in Nursing Science* 29, no. 4 (2006): 308–23.

Cohen, Marjorie Griffin. Review of *The Gendered Impacts of Liberalization: Towards 'Embedded Liberalism'?* edited by Shahra Razavi. *Feminist Economics* 16, no. 4 (2010): 211–15.

Cohen, Philip N., and Matt L. Huffman. "Individuals, Jobs, and Labor Markets: The Devaluation of Women's Work." *American Sociological Review* 68: 443–63.

Constable, Nicole. *Maid to Order in Hong Kong: Stories of Migrant Workers: Version 2.* Ithaca, NY: Cornell University Press, 2007.

Cook, T. G., ed. *Education and the Professions.* New York: Routledge, 1973.

Coole, Diane. "Women, Gender and Contract: Feminist Interpretations." In Kelly and Boucher, *Social Contract from Hobbes to Rawls*, 191–210. London: Routledge, 1994.

Cooper, Mary Carolyn. "Covenantal Relationships." *Advances in Nursing Science* 10, no. 4 (1988): 48–59.

Crenshaw, Kimberlé. "A Black Feminist Critique of Antidiscrimination Doctrine, Feminist Theory and Antiracist Politics." *University of Chicago Legal Forum* 140 (1989): 139–67.

———. "Mapping the Margins: Intersectionality, Identity Politics, and Violence against Women of Color." *Stanford Law Review* 43, no. 6 (July 1991): 1241–99.

Critchlow, Keith. *Quadrivium: The Four Classical Liberal Arts of Number, Geometry, Music, & Cosmology.* New York: Bloomsbury, 2010.

Crocker, David A. "Functioning and Capability: The Foundations of Sen's and Nussbaum's Development Ethic." *Political Theory* 20, no. 4 (1992): 584–612. Accessed May 6, 2015. http://www.jstor.org/stable/191970.

Cruess, Richard L., and Sylvia R. Cruess. "Expectations and Obligations: Professionalism and Medicine's Social Contract with Society." *Perspectives in Biology and Medicine* 51, no. 4 (2008): 579–98.

———. "Medicine's Social Contract with Society: Its Nature, Evolution, and Present State." In *Psychiatry's Contract with Society: Concepts, Controversies, and Consequences.* Edited by Dinesh Bhugra, Amit Malik, and George Ikkos, 123–46. Oxford, UK: Oxford University Press, 2010.

———. "Principles for Designing a Program for the Teaching and Learning of Professionalism at the Undergraduate Level." In Cruess, Cruess, and Steinert, *Teaching Medical Professionalism*, 73–92.

———. "Professionalism and Medicine's Social Contract." *Focus on Health Professional Education: A Multi-Professional Journal* 16, no. 1 (2014): 4–19.

———. "Updating the Hippocratic Oath to Include Medicine's Social Contract." *Medical Education* 48, no. 1 (2013): 95–100.

Cruess, Richard L., Sylvia R. Cruess, and Sharon E. Johnston. "Professionalism: An Ideal to Be Sustained." *Lancet* 356, no. 9224 (2000): 156–59.

———. "Renewing Professionalism." *Academic Medicine* 74, no. 8 (1999): 878–84.

Cruess, Richard L., Sylvia R. Cruess, and Yvonne Steinert, ed. *Teaching Medical Professionalism.* Cambridge, UK: Cambridge University Press, 2008.

Cruess, Sylvia R. 2006. "Professionalism and Medicine's Social Contract with Society." *Clinical Orthopaedics and Related Research* 449: 170–76.

Cruess, Sylvia R., Richard L. Cruess, and Yvonne Steinert. "Linking the Teaching of Professionalism to the Social Contract: A Call for Cultural Humility." *Medical Teacher* 32, no. 5 (2010): 357–59.

Czech, Brian. "Roll Over, Adam Smith: The 'New Economy Of Nature' Overlooks The Origins Of Money: A Review of *The New Economy of Nature: the Quest to Make Conservation Profitable* by Gretchen C. Daily and Katharine Ellison, eds." *BioScience* 53, no. 2 (2003): 180–83.

Daly, Herman E., and John B. Cobb. *For the Common Good: Redirecting the Economy toward Community, the Environment, and a Sustainable Future.* Boston: Beacon Press, 1991.

Davis, Fred, ed. *Nursing Profession: Five Sociological Essays.* New York: Wiley & Sons, 1966.

De Bettignies, Henri-Claude, and François Lépineux, ed. *Business, Globalization and the Common Good (Frontiers of Business Ethics).* New York: Verlag Peter Lang, 2009.

De Ridder-Symoens, Hilde. "Mobility." In Rüegg, *History of the University in Europe*, Vol. 1, 280–306.

Deere, Carmen. "The Feminization of Agriculture?: The Impact of Economic Restructuring in Rural Latin America." In Razavi, *Gendered Impacts of Liberalization Policies*, 99–127.

Donaldson, Thomas, and Thomas W. Dunfee. "Toward a Unified Conception of Business Ethics: Integrative Social Contracts Theory." *Academy of Management Review* 19, no. 2 (1994): 252–84. Accessed May 4, 2015. http://www.jstor.org/stable/258705.

Donley, Rosemary. "Revisiting the American Nurses Association's First Position on Education for Nurses." *Online Journal of Issues in Nursing* 7, no. 2 (2002), Manuscript 1. http://www.nursingworld.org/MainMenuCategories/ANAMarketplace/ANAPeriodicals/OJIN/TableofContents/Volume72002/No2May2002/RevisingPostiononEducation.html.

Dunning, John, ed. *Making Globalization Good: The Moral Challenges of Global Capitalism.* Oxford, UK: Oxford University Press, 2003.

Durkheim, Émile. *The Division of Labor in Society.* Translated by George Simpson. New York: The Free Press/Macmillan, 1933.

———. *On Morality and Society: Selected Writings.* Edited by Robert Neeley Bellah. Chicago: University of Chicago Press, 1975.

———. *Professional Ethics and Civic Morals.* Translated by Cornelia Brookfield. London: Routledge, 1957.

Duvvury, Nata, Vesna Malesevic, and Ernesto Vasquez de Aguila. "Introduction: Economic Crisis and Recovery: Gendered Impacts and Discourses." *Gender, Sexuality & Feminism* 1, no. 2 (December 2014): 1–4.

Dwyer, Rachel E. "The Care Economy? Gender, Economic Restructuring, and Job Polarization in the U.S. Labor Market." *American Sociological Review* 78, no. 3 (2013): 390–416.

Eckenwiler, Lisa. "Women on the Move: Long-Term Care, Migrant Women, and Global Justice." *International Journal of Feminist Approaches to Bioethics* 4.2 (December 2011): 1–31.

Edwards, Sebastian. "Structural Adjustment Policies in Highly Indebted Countries." In *Developing Country Debt and Economic Performance*, edited by Jeffrey Sachs,159–208. Chicago: University of Chicago, 1989.

Eisen, Robert. "'Lifnim Mi-Shurat Ha-Din' in Maimonides' 'Mishneh Torah.'" *Jewish Quarterly Review* 89, no. 3/4 (January 1999): 291–317.

Elshtain, Jean Bethke. *Public Man, Private Woman: Women in Social and Political Thought.* Oxford, UK: Robertson, 1982.

Etzioni, Amitai, ed. *The Semi-Professions and Their Organization; Teachers, Nurses, Social Workers.* New York: Collier-Macmillan, 1969.

Ewelukwa, Uchechukwu. "Post-Colonialism, Gender, Customary Injustice: Widows in African Societies." *Human Rights Quarterly* 24, no. 2 (2002): 424–86.

Fenstermacher, G., and J. R. Wiens, ed. *Yearbook of the National Society for the Study of Education.* Vol. 1. New York: The National Society for the Study of Education/Teachers' College Columbia, 2008.

Ferrall, Victor E. *Liberal Arts at the Brink.* Cambridge, MA: Harvard University Press, 2011.

Ferry, Michael. "Does Morality Demand Our Very Best? On Moral Prescriptions and the Line of Duty." *Philosophical Studies* 165, no. 2 (1 September 2013): 573–89.

Finkelman, Anita, and Carole Kenner. *Learning IOM: Implications of the Institute of Medicine Reports for Nursing Education.* Silver Spring, MD: American Nurses Association, 2012.

Fitzpatrick, Louise M. "Nursing." *Signs* 2.4 (1977): 818–34.

Flexner, Abraham. *Medical Education in the United States and Canada: A Report to the Carnegie Foundation for the Advancement of Teaching.* Boston, MA: Marymount Press, 1910.

Florovsky, Georges. *The Ways of Russian Theology.* Translated by Robert Nichols. Vols.1 and 2 Belmont, MA: Norland, 1979.

Fowler, Marsha D. M. *Central Themes in Russian Orthodox Christianity and the Concept of Health.* Moscow, Russia: Ministry of Health, Republic of Russia, 1994.

———. *Guide to the Code of Ethics for Nurses: Development, Interpretation, and Application.* 2nd ed. Silver Spring, MD: American Nurses Association, 2015.

———. ed. *Guide to the Code of Ethics for Nurses: Interpretation and Application.* Silver Spring, MD: American Nurses Association, 2008.

———. "Is Occupational Labor a Spiritual Endeavor." *Park Ridge Center Bulletin*, Winter, September 2001: 5–6.

———. "Professional Associations, Ethics and Society." *Oncology Nursing Forum* 20, no. 10, supplement to Nov/Dec 1993 issue:13–19.

———. "Social Ethics and Nursing." In Chaska, *Nursing Profession*, 24–31.

———. "Social Ethics and the Role of Professional Associations." In *New Nurses for a New Russia.* Moscow: Ministry of Health, Republic of Russia, 1994.

———. "Spirituality, Faith, and Nursing Practice." In *New Nurses for a New Russia.* Moscow: Ministry of Health, Republic of Russia, 1994.

Fowler, Marsha D. M., Sheryl Reimer Kirkham, Rick Sawatzky, and Elizabeth Johnston Taylor, ed. *Religion, Religious Ethics and Nursing.* New York: Springer Publishing Company, 2011.

Francis, Becky, and John Humphreys. "Rationalisation and Professionalisation: A Comparison of the Transfer of Registered Nurse Education to Higher Education in Australia and the UK." *Comparative Education* 35 (1999): 81–96. Accessed May 6, 2015. http://www.jstor.org/stable/3099468.

Freidson, Eliot. *Professional Dominance: The Social Structure of Medical Care (Pbk).* New Brunswick, NJ: Atherton Press/Aldine Publishing, 1970.

———. *Professional Powers: A Study of the Institutionalization of Formal Knowledge.* 2nd ed. Chicago: University Of Chicago Press, 1988.

———. *Professionalism, the Third Logic: On the Practice of Knowledge.* Chicago: University of Chicago Press, 2001.

Froth, Thomas. "Nurses, medical records and the killing of sick persons before, during, and after the Nazi regime in Germany." *Nursing Inquiry* 20, no. 2 (2013): 92–100.

———. "Understanding 'Caring' through Biopolitics: The Case of Nurses under the Nazi Regime." *Nursing Philosophy* 14, no. 4 (2013): 284–94.

Fry, Sara T. "Accountability in Research." *Advances in Nursing Science* 4, no. 1 (1981): 1–13.

———. "Nursing Ethics." In *Handbook of Bioethics, Philosophy and Medicine*, 489–505. Netherlands: Springer/Kluwer, 2004.

———. "The Role of Caring in a Theory of Nursing Ethics." *Hypatia* 4, no. 2 (1989): 87–103.

———. "Toward a Theory of Nursing Ethics." *Advances in Nursing Science* 11, no. 4 (1989): 9–22.

Gardner, Clinton E. "Justice, Virtue, and Law." *Journal of Law and Religion* 2, no. 2 (1984): 393–412.

Garner, Bryan A., ed. *Black's Law Dictionary*. Eagan, MN: Thomson West Publishing Co, 2014.

Geison, Gerald L., ed. *Professions and Professional Ideologies in America*. Chapel Hill, NC: University of North Carolina Press, 1984.

George, Susan. *A Fate Worse Than Debt*. New York: Grove Weidenfeld, 1990.

Gilligan, Carol. *In a Different Voice: Psychological Theory and Women's Development*. Cambridge, MA: Harvard University Press, 1982.

Gilman, J. E. "Compassion and Public Covenant: Christian Faith in Public Life." *Journal of Church and State* 36, no. 4 (1994): 747–71.

Glazer, Nona Y. "'Between a Rock and a Hard Place': Women's Professional Organizations in Nursing and Class, Racial, and Ethnic Inequalities." *Gender and Society* 5, no. 3 (September 1991): 351–72.

Gordon, Robert J. "Does the 'New Economy' Measure up to the Great Inventions of the Past?" *Journal of Economic Perspectives* 14, no. 4 (2000): 49–74.

Greenwood, Ernest. "Attributes of a Profession." *Social Work* 2, no. 3 (1957): 45–55.

Gregory, Alex. "A Very Good Reason to Reject the Buck-Passing Account." *Australasian Journal of Philosophy* 92, no. 2 (2013): 287–303.

Groce, Nora Ellen, and Reshma Trasi. "Rape of Individuals with Disability: AIDS and the Folk Belief of Virgin Cleansing." *Lancet* 363, no. 9422 (2004): 1663–64.

Guevara, Daniel. "The Impossibility of Supererogation in Kant's Moral Theory." *Philosophy and Phenomenological Research* 59, no. 3 (September 1999): 593–624.

Hafferty, Frederic William. "Professionalism and the Socialization of Medical Students." In Cruess, Cruess, and Steinert, *Teaching Medical Professionalism*, 53–70.

Haigh, Martin. "From Internationalisation to Education for Global Citizenship: A Multi-Layered History." *Higher Education Quarterly* 68, no. 1 (2014): 6–27.

Hall, Robert T. "Emile Durkheim on Business and Professional Ethics." *Business and Professional Ethics Journal* 2, no. 1 (1982): 51–60.

Hallett, Christine. *Women and Social Policy: An Introduction*. London: Prentice Hall/Harvester Wheatsheaf in association with SPA Social Policy Association, 1995.

Hampton, Jean. "Feminist Contractarianism." In Antony and Witt, *Mind of One's Own*, 337–68.

———. *Hobbes and the Social Contract Tradition*. Cambridge, UK: Cambridge University Press, 1988.

———. "Two Faces of Contractarian Thought." In Vallentyne, *Contractarianism and Rational Choice*, 31–55.

Hamric, Ann B. "A Case Study of Moral Distress." *Journal of Hospice & Palliative Nursing* 16, no. 8 (2014): 457–63.

———. "Empirical Research on Moral Distress: Issues, Challenges, and Opportunities." *HEC Forum* 24, no. 1 (March 2012): 39–49.

———. "Moral Distress and Nurse-Physician Relationships." *Virtual Mentor* 12, no. 1 (2010): 6–11.

Hatch, Nathan O., ed. *The Professions in American History*. Notre Dame, IN: University of Notre Dame Press, 1988.

Held, Virginia. *Feminist Morality: Transforming Culture, Society, and Politics*. Chicago: University of Chicago Press, 1993.

———. "Noncontractual Society: A Feminist View." Edited by M. P. Haren and Kai Nielsen. *Science, Morality and Feminist Theory* 13, Supplement (1 December 1987): 111–37.

Helmstadter, Carol. "Shifting Boundaries: Religion, Medicine, Nursing and Domestic Service in Mid-Nineteenth-Century Britain." *Nursing Inquiry* 16: 133–43.

Helmstadter, Carol, and Judith Godden. "Nursing Before Nightingale, 1815–1899." *Nursing History Review* 21, no. 1 (2013): 122–54.

Hill, T. Patrick. "Health Care: A Social Contract in Transition." *Social Science & Medicine* 43, no. 5 (1996): 783–89.

Hill, Thomas E., and Adam Cureton. "Supererogation." In *International Encyclopedia of Ethics*, edited by Hugh LaFollette, page range. Location: Wiley-Blackwell, 2013.

Hill, Jr., Thomas E. "And on Imperfect Duty and Supererogation." *Kant-Studien* 62 (1971): 55–76.

Hobbes, Thomas. *Thomas Hobbes: Leviathan.* Edited by Richard Tuck. Cambridge, UK: Cambridge University Press, 1991.

Holmboe, Eric, and Elizabeth Bernabeo. "The 'Special Obligations' of the Modern Hippocratic Oath for 21st Century Medicine". *Medical Education* 48, no. 1 (2013): 87–94.

Horkheimer, Max. *Critical Theory: Selected Essays.* New York: Seabury, 1982.

Hunter, Anita, Lynda Wilson, Marcia Stanhope, Barbara Hatcher, Marianne Hattar, DeAnne Hilfinger K. Messias, and Dorothy Powell. "Global Health Diplomacy: An Integrative Review of the Literature and Implications for Nursing." *Nursing Outlook* 61, no. 2 (2013): 85–92.

Hurd, Richard, ed. *The Works of the Right Honorable Joseph Addison in 6 Volumes.* Vol. 2. Covent Garden, UK: Henry G. Bohn, 1856.

International Council of Nurses. *The ICN Code of Ethics for Nurses.* Geneva: ICN, 2000.

International Labor Organization. 2004. "Bureau of Statistics, Work Unit of the Policy Integration Department." Last modified October 4, 2004. Accessed May 6, 2015. http://www.ilo.org/public/english/bureau/stat/isco/intro.htm.

Jackson, John Archer. *Professions and Professionalization.* Volume 3, *Sociological Studies.* London: Cambridge University Press, 1971.

Jackson, Robert. *The Global Covenant: Human Conduct in a World of States.* Oxford, UK: Oxford University Press, 2000.

Jennings, Bruce. "Beyond the Social Contract of Consumption: Democratic Governance in the Post-Carbon Era." *Critical Policy Studies* 4, no. 3 (2010): 222–33.

John, Rawls. *A Theory of Justice.* Cambridge, MA: Belknap Press of Harvard Univ. Press, 1972.

Johnson, Benjamin. *Steal This University: The Rise of the Corporate University and the Academic Labor Movement.* Edited by Patrick Kavanaugh and Kevin Mattson. New York: Routledge, 2003.

Johnson, Terence James. *Professions and Power.* London: Macmillan, 1972.

Johri, Mira, Ryoa Chung, Angus Dawson, and Ted Schrecker. "Global Health and National Borders: The Ethics of Foreign Aid in a Time of Financial Crisis." *Globalization and Health* 8, no. 19 (June 2012): 1–10. doi: 10.1186/1744-8603-8-19.

Jowett, Benjamin, and Albert A. Anderson. *Plato's Euthyphro, Apology, Crito, Phaedo: Theater of the Mind.* Millis, MA: Agora Publications, 2005.

Katz, Jay. "Human Sacrifice and Human Experimentation: Reflections at Nuremberg." *Yale Journal of International Law* 22, no. 401 (1997): 401–18.

———. "The Nuremberg Code, German Law, and Prominent Physician-Thinkers-Reply." *Journal of the American Medical Association* 277, no. 9 (1997): 709–10.

———. "The Nuremberg Code and the Nuremberg Trial. A Reappraisal." *Journal of the American Medical Association* 276, no. 20 (1996): 1662–66.

Keck, Margaret E., and K. Sikkink. *Activists Beyond Borders*. Ithaca, NY: Cornell University Press, 1998.

Keck, Margaret E. *Activistas Sin Fronteras*. México, D.F: Siglo Veintiuno Editores, 2000.

Kelly, Paul and David Boucher, ed. *The Social Contract from Hobbes to Rawls*. New York: Taylor & Francis, 1994.

Kim, ChangHwan, and Arthur Sakamoto. "The Rise of Intra-Occupational Wage Inequality in the United States, 1983 to 2002." *American Sociological Review* 73, no. 1 (2008): 129–57. Accessed May 6, 2015. doi: 10.1177/000312240807300107.

Kittay, Eva, and Ellen K. Feder, ed. *The Subject of Care: Feminist Perspectives on Dependency*. Lanham, MD: Rowman & Littlefield Publishers, 2003.

Kittay, Eva Feder, Bruce Jennings, and Angela A. Wasunna. "Dependency, Difference and the Global Ethic of Longterm Care." *Journal of Political Philosophy* 13, no. 4 (2005): 443–69.

Klot, Jennifer F., and Vinh-Kim Nguyen, ed. *The Fourth Wave: Violence, Gender, Culture & HIV in the 21st Century*. Paris: UNESCO, 2011.

Kraut, Richard. *Socrates and the State*. Princeton, NJ: Princeton University Press, 1992.

Kruks, Sonia, Tamsin E. Lorraine, Elizabeth Fox-Genovese, Mary Lyndon-Shanley, and Carol Pateman. "Gender, Identity, and the Production of Meaning." *American Political Science Review* 86, no. 1 (1992): 216–18.

Kurlander, Jacob E., Karine Morin, and Matthew K. Wynia. "The Social-Contract Model of Professionalism: Baby or Bath Water?" *American Journal of Bioethics* 4, no. 2 (2004): 33–36.

Küng, Hans. "An Ethical Framework for the Global Market Economy." In Dunning, *Making Globalization Good*, 145–58.

Lagerwey, Mary. "Nursing Ethics at Hadamar." *Qualitative Health Research* 9, no. 6 (November 1999): 759–72.

Laiho, Anne. "Academisation of Nursing Education in the Nordic Countries." *Higher Education* 60, no. 6 (December 2010): 641–56.

Laird, Sam, and Julio Nogués. "Trade Policies and the Highly Indebted Countries." *World Bank Economic Review* 3, no. 2 (1989): 241–61.

Larson, Magali Sarfatti. *The Rise of Professionalism: A Sociological Analysis*. Berkeley: University of California Press, 1980.

Lavengood, Lawrence G. Review of *Ties That Bind: A Social Contracts Approach to Business Ethics* by Thomas Donaldson and Thomas W. Dunfee. *Ethics* 111, no. 3 (2001): 627–30.

Lee, Sidney S. "Health Policy, a Social Contract: A Comparison of the United States and Canada." *Journal of Public Health Policy* 3, no. 3 (September 1982): 293–301.

Locke, John. *Locke: Two Treatises of Government*. Edited by Peter Laslett. Cambridge, UK: Cambridge University Press, 1967.

Lomasky, Loren E. "Contract, Covenant, Constitution." *Social Philosophy and Policy* 28, no. 01 (2010): 50–71.

Lossky, Vladimir. *Mystical Theology of the Eastern Church*. Crestwood, NY: St. Vladimir's Seminary Press, 1976.

———. *Orthodox Theology: An Introduction*. Crestwood, NY: St. Vladimir's Seminary Press, 1989.

Lowrance, William O. *Of Acceptable Risk: Science and the Determination of Safety*. Los Altos, CA: William Kaufmann, 1976.

Lundmark, M. "Vocation in Theology-Based Nursing Theories." *Nursing Ethics* 14, no. 6 (2007): 767–80.

MacDonald, Keith M. *The Sociology of the Professions.* Thousand Oaks, CA: Sage Publications, 1995.

Macpherson, Crawford Brough. *The Political Theory of Possessive Individualism: Hobbes to Locke.* Oxford, UK: Clarendon Press, 1964.

Malm, Heidi, Thomas May, Leslie P. Francis, Saad B. Omer, Daniel A. Salmon, and Robert Hood. "Ethics, Pandemics, and the Duty to Treat." *American Journal of Bioethics* 8, no. 8 (2008): 4–19.

Marshall, Jill. Review of *The Classic Social Contractarians: Critical Perspectives from Contemporary Feminist Philosophy and Law* by Janice Richardson. *Feminist Legal Studies* 18, no. 1 (21 April 2010): 109–12.

Marshall, T. H. "The Recent History of Professionalism in Relation to Social Structure and Social Policy." *Canadian Journal of Economics and Political Science* 5, no. 3 (1939): 325–40.

Masters, Roger D. "Is Contract an Adequate Basis for Medical Ethics?" *Hastings Center Report* 5, no. 6 (1975): 24–28.

Matsuda, Mari. "Liberal Jurisprudence and Abstracted Visions of Human Nature: A Feminist Critique of Rawls' Theory of Justice." *New Mexico Law Review* 16, no. 3 (1986): 613–30.

May, William F. "Code, Covenant, Contract, or Philanthropy." *Hastings Center Report* 5, no. 6 (December 1975): 29–38.

McDonald, Allan J, and James R. Hansen. *Truth, Lies, and O-Rings: Inside the Space Shuttle Challenger Disaster.* Gainesville: University Press of Florida, 2009.

McDonald, Lynn, ed. *Florence Nightingale: Extending Nursing.* Vol. 13 of the *Collected Works of Florence Nightingale.* Ontario: Wilfrid Laurier University Press, 2006.

———, ed. *Florence Nightingale's Theology: Essays, Letters and Journal Notes.* Vol. 3 of the *Collected Works of Florence Nightingale.* Ontario: Wilfrid Laurier University Press, 2002.

McHugh, Matthew D., Margo Brooks Carthon, Douglas M. Sloane, Evan Wu, Lesly Kelly, and Linda H. Aiken. "Impact of Nurse Staffing Mandates on Safety-Net Hospitals: Lessons from California." *Milbank Quarterly* 90, no. 1 (March 2012): 160–86.

McKie, Andrew. "'The Demolition of a Man': Lessons from Holocaust Literature for the Teaching of Nursing Ethics." *Nursing Ethics* 11, no. 2 (2004): 138–4.

Meel, B L. "The Myth of Child Rape as a Cure for HIV/AIDS in Transkei." *Medicine, Science and the Law* 43, no. 1 (2003): 85–88.

Melden, Abraham I., ed. *Essays Moral Philosophy.* Seattle: University of Washington Press, 1967.

Melosh, Barbara. *The Physician's Hand: Work Culture and Conflict in American Nursing.* Philadelphia: Temple University Press, 1982.

———. "'Skilled Hands, Cool Heads, and Warm Hearts': Nurses and Nursing 1920–1960." PhD diss., Brown University, 1979.

Menand, Louis. *The Marketplace of Ideas: Reform and Resistance in the American University.* Issues of Our Time Series. New York: W. W. Norton & Company, 2010.

Mill, John Stuart. *On Liberty and Other Essays.* Edited by John Gray. New York: Oxford University Press, 1991.

Millerson, Geoffrey. "Education in the Professions." In Cook, *Education and the Professions*, 1–18.

Mills, Charles W. *The Racial Contract.* Ithaca, NY: Cornell University Press, 2014.

Mooney, Mary, and Louise Nolan. "A Critique of Freire's Perspective on Critical Social Theory in Nursing Education." *Nurse Education Today* 26, no. 3 (2006): 240–44.

Mount, Eric. *Covenant, Community, and the Common Good.* Cleveland, OH: United Church Press, 1999.

National Research Council, and Center for Education. *The Knowledge Economy and Postsecondary Education: Report of a Workshop.* Edited by Patricia Albjerg Graham. Washington, DC: National Academies Press, 2002.

Nayo, Lydia A., Martha Minow, and Mari J. Matsuda. "In Search of Common Ground." *Women's Review of Books* 15, no. 5 (February 1998): 9.

Nelson, Sioban, and Suzanne Gordon, ed. *The Complexities of Care: Nursing Reconsidered.* Ithaca, NY: ILR Press of Cornell University Press, 2006.

Niebuhr, Richard. "The Idea of Covenant and American Democracy." *Church History* 23, no. 2 (1954): 126–35.

Nightingale, Florence. *Florence Nightingale to Her Nurses: A Selection from Miss Nightingale's Addresses to Probationers and Nurses of the Nightingale School at St. Thomas's Hospital.* London: Macmillan, 1914.

Nordhaus, William D. "Productivity Growth and the New Economy: Brookings Papers on Economic Activity." *National Bureau of Economic Research* 8096 (January 2001): 1–48.

Norrish, Barbara R., and Thomas G. Rundall. "Hospital Restructuring and the Work of Registered Nurses." *Milbank Quarterly* 79, no. 1 (2001): 55–79.

Norton, R. D. *Creating the New Economy: The Entrepreneur and the U. S. Resurgence.* Cheltenham, UK: Edward Elgar Publishing, 2001.

Noyes, Clara D. "American Nurses' Memorial, Bordeaux, France." *American Journal of Nursing* 24, no. 3 (1923): 192.

Nussbaum, Martha. "Capabilities as Fundamental Entitlements: Sen and Social Justice." *Feminist Economics* 9, no. 2–3 (2003): 33–59.

———. *Creating Capabilities: The Human Development Approach.* Cambridge, MA: Belknap Press of Harvard University Press, 2011.

———. *Cultivating Humanity: A Classical Defense of Reform in Liberal Education.* Cambridge, MA: Harvard University Press, 1998.

———. *Frontiers of Justice: Disability, Nationality, Species Membership.* Cambridge, MA: Belknap Press of Harvard University Press, 2007.

———. *Women and Human Development: The Capabilities Approach.* Cambridge, MA: Cambridge University Press, 2001.

Okin, Susan Moller. *Justice, Gender, and the Family.* New York: Basic Books, 1989.

Olson, Jonas. "Buck-Passing and the Wrong Kind of Reasons." *Philosophical Quarterly* 54, no. 215 (April 2004): 295–300.

O'Neil, Robert. *Academic Freedom in a Wired World: Political Extremism, and the University.* Vol. 46. Cambridge, MA: Harvard University Press, 2008.

Ooms, Gorik, Moses Mulumba, Rachel Hammonds, Abdul Latif Laila, Attiya Waris, and Lisa Forman. "A Global Social Contract to Reduce Maternal Mortality: The Human Rights Arguments and the Case of Uganda." *Reproductive Health Matters* 21, no. 42 (2013): 129–38.

Ottati, Douglas F. "Reformed Theology, Revelation, and Particularity: John Calvin and H. Richard Niebuhr." *CrossCurrents* 59, no. 2 (2009): 127–43.

Page, B. B. "Who Owns the Professions?" *Hastings Center Report* 5, no. 5 (1975): 7–8.

Pappworth, M. H. *Human Guinea Pigs: Experimentation on Man.* London: Routledge & Keagan, 1967.

———. "'Human Guinea Pigs'—a History." *British Medical Journal* 301, no. 6766 (1990): 1456–60.

Parreñas, Rhacel Salazar, and Eileen Boris, ed. *Intimate Labors: Cultures, Technologies, and the Politics of Care*. Stanford, CA: Stanford University Press, 2010.

Parsons, Sara E. "Ethics: The Probationer." *American Journal of Nursing* 16, no. 10 (1916): 975–80.

Parsons, Talcott. "The Professions and Social Structure." *Social Forces* 17, no. 4 (May 1939): 457–67.

Partington, Angela, ed. *The Oxford Dictionary of Quotations*. Oxford, UK: Oxford University Press, 1992.

Pateman, Carole. "'God Hath Ordained to Man a Helper': Hobbes, Patriarchy and Conjugal Rights." *British Journal of Political Science* 19, no. 4 (1991): 445–63.

———. "Myth, History, and Democracy: Alien Reflections." *Social Text* 56 (1998): 53–56.

———. *Participation and Democratic Theory (Structural Analysis in the Social Sciences)*. Cambridge, UK: Cambridge University Press, 1976.

———. "Political Culture, Political Structure and Political Change." *British Journal of Political Science* 1, no. 3 (July 1971): 291–305.

———. *The Problem of Political Obligation: A Critical Analysis of Liberal Theory*. Berkeley: University of California Press, 1985.

———. *The Sexual Contract*. Stanford: Stanford University Press, 1988.

———. "Women and Consent." *Political Theory* 8, no. 2 (May 1980): 149–68.

Pateman, Carole, Nancy J. Hirschmann, and Bingham G. Powell. "Political Obligation, Freedom and Feminism." *American Political Science Review* 86, no. 1 (March 1992): 179–88.

Peck, Harvey W. "The New Economy and the Machine." *Social Forces* 22, no. 1 (1943): 47–55.

Pellegrino, Edmund D., and David C. Thomasma. *For the Patient's Good: The Restoration of Beneficence in Health Care*. New York: Oxford University Press, 1988.

———. *A Philosophical Basis of Medical Practice*. New York: Oxford University Press, 1981.

Perelman, Chaim, L. Olbrechts-Tyteca, John Wilkinson, and Purcell Weaver. *The New Rhetoric: A Treatise on Argumentation*. Translated by John Wilkinson and Purcell Weaver. Notre Dame, IN: University of Notre Dame Press, 1973.

Perrons, Diane, Colette Fagan, Linda McDowell, Kath Ray, and Kevin Ward, ed. *Gender Divisions And Working Time In The New Economy Changing Patterns of Work, Care and Public Policy in Europe and North America*. Cheltenham, UK: Edward Elgar Publishing, 2006.

Perrucci, Robert, and Carolyn C. Perrucci, ed. *The Transformation of Work in the New Economy: Sociological Readings*. 2nd ed. Los Angeles: Roxbury Publishing, 2007.

Peter, Elizabeth, and Joan Liaschenko. "Moral Distress Reexamined: A Feminist Interpretation of Nurses' Identities, Relationships, and Responsibilities." *Journal of Bioethical Inquiry* 10, no. 3 (1 October 2013): 337–45.

Pham, Milan Trinh. Review of *Where Is Your Body? And Other Essays on Race, Gender, and the Law* by Mari J. Matsuda. *Contemporary Sociology* 27, no. 6 (1998): 650.

Plato. *Republic*. Translated by Robin Waterfield. New York: Oxford University Press, 1993.

"The Policy Roots of Economic Crisis and Poverty." Report prepared by the Structural Adjustment Participatory Review International Network in Washington, DC, April 2002. http://www.saprin.org/SAPRIN_Findings.pdf.

Powell, Walter. *Private Action and the Public Good*. Edited by Walter W. Powell and Elisabeth S. Clemens. New Haven, CT: Yale University Press, 1998.

Ramsey, Paul. *The Patient as Person: Explorations in Medical Ethics*. New Haven, CT: Yale University Press, 1970.

Rashdall, Hastings, Frederick M. Powicke, and A. B. Emden. *The Universities of Europe in the Middle Ages.* Vol. 3, *English Universities - Student Life.* Oxford: Clarendon Press, 1936.

Raskin, Marcus G. *Common Good: Its Politics, Policies and Philosophy.* New York: Routledge & Kegan Paul Books, 1986.

Razavi, Shahra, ed. *The Gendered Impacts of Liberalization: Towards 'Embedded Liberalism'?* New York: Routledge, 2011.

Reeves, Scott, Mary van Soeren, Kathleen MacMillan, and Merrick Zwarenstein. "Medicine and Nursing: A Social Contract to Improve Collaboration and Patient-Centred Care?" *Journal of Interprofessional Care* 27, no. 6 (2013): 441–42.

Rehmann-Sutter, Christoph, Marcus Dýwell, and Dietmar Mieth. *Bioethics in Cultural Contexts: Reflections on Methods and Finitude.* New York: Springer-Verlag, 2006.

Reid, Lynette. "Medical Professionalism and the Social Contract." *Perspectives in Biology and Medicine* 54, no. 4 (2011): 455–69.

Reilly, Richard. *Ethics of Compassion: Bridging Ethical Theory and Religious Moral Discourse.* n.p.: Lexington Books, 2010.

Reimer-Kirkham, Sheryl. "Nursing Research on Religion and Spirituality Through a Social Justice Lens." *Advances in Nursing Science* 37, no. 3 (2014): 249–57.

Reiser, Stanley Joel. "Creating a Medical Profession in the United States: The First Code of Ethics of the American Medical Association." In *The Codification of Medical Morality: Historical and Philosophical Studies of the Formalization of Western Medical Morality in the Eighteenth and Nineteenth Centuries,* Vol. 2, *Anglo-American Medical Ethics and Medical Jurisprudence in the Nineteenth Century,* edited by Robert Baker, 89–103. New York: Springer, 1995.

Reiser, Stanley Joel, and Ruth E. Bulger. "The Social Responsibilities of Biological Scientists." *Science and Engineering Ethics* 3, no. 2 (1 June 1997): 137–43.

Reynolds, Ruth. "Civics and Citizenship Education in Its Global Context: The Complexity of Global Citizenship Dialogues." *Education Sciences* 2, no. 4 (2012): 190–92.

Richardson, Henry S. "Rawlsian Social-Contract Theory and the Severely Disabled." *Journal of Ethics* 10, no. 4 (22 January 2007): 419–62.

Richardson, Janice. "Contemporary Feminist Perspectives on Social Contract Theory." *Ratio Juris* 20, no. 3 (2007): 402–23.

Rogers, Jamie, and Ursula A. Kelly. "Feminist Intersectionality: Bringing Social Justice to Health Disparities Research." *Nursing Ethics* 18, no. 3 (2011): 397–407.

Rollins, Joe. "PS: Political Science, Political Sex." *PS: Political Science and Politics* 44, no. 1 (January 2011): 27–30.

Roth, Michael S. *Beyond the University: Why Liberal Education Matters.* New Haven, CT: Yale University Press, 2014.

Rousseau, Jean-Jacques. *Basic Political Writings: Discourse on the Sciences and the Arts, Discourse on the Origin of Inequality, Discourse on Political Economy, On the Social Contract, The State of War.* 2nd ed. Edited and translated by David Wooten, and Donald A. Cress. Indianapolis: Hackett Publishing Company, 2012.

Rowden, Rick. *The Deadly Ideas of Neoliberalism: How the IMF Has Undermined Public Health and the Fight against AIDS.* London: Zed Books, 2009.

Rowland, Richard. "Why Pass Every Buck? On Skorupsk's Buck-Passing Account of Normativity." *Ratio* 24, no. 3 (2011): 340–48.

Russell, Anthony. *The Clerical Profession.* London: SPCK Publishing, 1980.

Rüegg, Walter, ed. *A History of the University in Europe.* Vol. 1, *Universities in the Middle Ages.* Edited by Hilde de Ridder-Symoens. Cambridge, UK: Cambridge University Press, 1992.

———, ed. *A History of the University in Europe*. Vol. 3, *Universities in the Nineteenth and Early Twentieth Centuries (1800–1945)*. Cambridge, UK: Cambridge University Press, 1992.

Sacks, Jonathan. "Global Covenant: A Jewish Perspective on Globalization." In Dunning, *Making Globalization Good*, 210–31.

Saks, Mike. "Defining a Profession: The Role of Knowledge and Expertise." *Professions & Professionalism* 2 (June 2010): 1–10.

Salami, Bukola, and Sioban Nelson. "The Downward Occupational Mobility of Internationally Educated Nurses to Domestic Workers." *Nursing Inquiry* 21, no. 2 (2013): 153–61.

Sample, Ruth. "Why Feminist Contractarianism?" *Journal of Social Philosophy* 33, no. 2 (2002): 257–81.

Schall, Mary Beth, and Jeanne Flannery. "Directions for Curricular Change: The 1980 and 1995 American Nurses Association's Policy Statements." *Nurse Educator* 25, no. 1 (2000): 17–18.

Scharton, Kathryn. "Reforming Nurses: Historicizing the Carnegie Foundation's Report on Educating Nurses." *Nursing History Review* 21, no. 1 (2013): 97–108.

Schrecker, Ellen. "Academic Freedom in the Corporate University." *Radical Teacher*, no. 93 (2012): 38–45.

———. *The Lost Soul of Higher Education: Corporatization, the Assault on Academic Freedom, and the End of the American University*. New York: The New Press, 2010.

Shah, Anup. "Structural Adjustment—a Major Cause of Poverty." *Global Issues*, March 24, 2013. http://www.globalissues.org/article/3/structural-adjustment-a-major-cause-of-poverty.

Sheahan, Dorothy Alice. "The Social Origins of American Nursing and Its Movement into the University: A Microscopic Approach." PhD diss., New York University, 1980.

Silva, Mary Cipriano. "The American Nurses' Association's Position Statement on Nursing and Social Policy: Philosophical and Ethical Dimensions." *Journal of Advanced Nursing* 8, no. 2 (1983): 147–51.

Silvers, Anita, and Leslie Pickering Francis. "Justice through Trust: Disability and the 'Outlier Problem' in Social Contract Theory." *Ethics* 116, no. 1 (October 2005): 40–76.

Sim, Julius. "Nursing Research: Is There an Obligation on Subjects to Participate?" *Journal of Advanced Nursing* 16, no. 11 (1991): 1284–89.

Sinha, Michael S. "Rousseau at the Roundtable—The Social Contract and the Physician's Responsibility to Society." *Virtual Mentor* 13, no. 10 (2011): 703–6.

Slaughter, Sheila, and Gary Rhoades. "From 'Endless Frontier' to 'Basic Science for Use': Social Contracts between Science and Society." *Science, Technology, & Human Values* 30, no. 4 (2005): 536–72.

Sleicher, M.N. "Nursing Is Not a Profession." *Nursing and Health Care* 2, no. 4 (April 1981): 186–92.

Smith, Pam, and Maureen Mackintosh. "Profession, Market and Class: Nurse Migration and the Remaking of Division and Disadvantage." *Journal of Clinical Nursing* 16, no. 12 (2007): 2213–20.

Spitzer, Denise L. "In Visible Bodies: Minority Women, Nurses, Time, and the New Economy of Care." *Medical Anthropology Quarterly* 18, no. 4 (December 2004): 490–508.

Steeman, Theodore M. "Durkheim's Professional Ethics." *Journal for the Scientific Study of Religion* 2, no. 2 (1963): 163–81.

Stenberg, Marjorie Jones. "Ethics as a Component of Nursing Education." *Advances in Nursing Science* 1, no. 3 (1979): 53–62.

Styles, Margretta M. *On Nursing: Toward a New Endowment*. St. Louis, MO: C. V. Mosby, 1982.

Suikkanen, Jussi. "Buck-Passing Accounts of Value." *Philosophy Compass* 4, no. 5 (2009): 768–79.

Sullivan, William M., and Lee S. Shulman. *Work and Integrity: The Crisis and Promise of Professionalism in America: The Carnegie Foundation for the Advancement of Teaching.* 2nd ed. San Francisco: Jossey-Bass, 2004.

Sullivan, William M., and Patricia Benner. "Challenges to Professionalism: Work Integrity and the Call to Renew and Strengthen the Social Contract of the Professions." *American Journal of Critical Care* 14, no. 1 (January 2005): 78–80.

Sullivan, William M., and Will Kymlicka. "International Covenant on Civil and Political Rights." In *Religious and Secular Perspectives,* edited by William Sullivan and Will Kymlicka, 219–28. Cambridge, UK: Cambridge University Press, 2007.

Sullivan, William M. "Can Professionalism Still Be a Viable Ethic?" *Good Society* 13, no. 1 (2004): 15–20.

———. *Work and Integrity: The Crisis and Promise of Professionalism in America.* 2nd ed. San Francisco: Jossey-Bass, 2005.

Sunshine, Fabio Grobart, and Mariana Ortega Breña. "Science and Technology in the United States: Hegemony Under Fire." *Latin American Perspectives* 34, no. 1 (January 2007): 39–45.

Sweet, Stephen A., and Peter Meiksins. *Changing Contours of Work: Jobs and Opportunities in the New Economy.* 2nd ed. Thousand Oaks, CA: SAGE, 2007.

Tawil, Sobhi. "Education for 'Global Citizenship': A Framework for Discussion." UNESCO Education Research and Foresight Working Papers 7, 2013.http://www.unesco.org/new/fileadmin/MULTIMEDIA/HQ/ED/pdf/PaperN7EducforGlobalCitizenship.pdf.

Thorne, Sally E. "Nursing Education: Key Issues for the 21st Century." *Nurse Education in Practice* 6, no. 6 (2006): 306–13.

Tilgher, Adriano. *Homo Faber: Work through the Ages.* Washington, DC: Regnery Publishing, 1958.

Tronto, Joan C. *Moral Boundaries: A Political Argument for an Ethic of Care.* New York: Taylor & Francis, 1994.

Tyson, Scott. "Centralized Coercive Force and the Political Foundations of Centralized Authority." *Social Science Research Network Electronic Journal,* January 2015: 1–47.

U.S. Office of Personnel Management. US Government Handbook of Occupational Groups and Families. Washington, DC: United States Government Printing Office, 2009. http://www.opm.gov/policy-data-oversight/classification-qualifications/classifying-general-schedule-positions/occupationalhandbook.pdf.

Ulrich, Connie M., Ann B. Hamric, and Christine Grady. "Moral Distress: A Growing Problem in the Health Professions?" *Hastings Center Report* 40, no. 1 (2010): 20–22.

Urmson, James Opie. "Saints and Heroes." In Melden, *Essays in Moral Philosophy,* 198–216.

Vallee, Gerard, ed. *Florence Nightingale on Mysticism and Eastern Religions.* Vol. 4 of the *Collected Works of Florence Nightingale.* Ontario: Wilfrid Laurier University Press, 2006.

Van der Merwe, Anita S. "The Power of Women as Nurses in South Africa." *Journal of Advanced Nursing* 30 (1999): 1272–79.

Vallentyne, Peter, ed. *Contractarianism and Rational Choice: Essays on David Gauthier's Morals by Agreement.* New York: Cambridge University Press, 1991.

Van Herk, Kimberley A, Dawn Smith, and Caroline Andrew. "Examining Our Privileges and Oppressions: Incorporating an Intersectionality Paradigm into Nursing." *Nursing Inquiry* 18, no. 1 (2011): 29–39.

Van Steenbergen, Bart, ed. *The Condition of Citizenship*. Thousand Oaks, CA: SAGE Publications, 1994.

Vaux, Kenneth. *Powers That Make Us Human: Foundations of Medical Ethics*. Chicago: University of Illinois Press, 1986.

Veatch, Robert. *The Patient as Partner: A Theory of Human-Experimentation Ethics*. Indianapolis: Indiana University Press, 1987.

Vollmer, Howard, and Donald Mills. *Professionalization*. Englewood Cliffs, NJ: Prentice-Hall, 1966.

Walby, Sylvia. "Analyzing Social Inequality in the Twenty-First Century: Globalization and Modernity Restructure Inequality." *Contemporary Sociology* 29, no. 6 (November 2000): 813–18.

Walkerdine, Valerie. "Workers in the New Economy: Transformation as Border Crossing." *Ethos* 34, no. 1 (March 2006): 10–41.

Weaver, Karol. "Review Essay: Reproduction in the United States." *Nursing History Review* 21, no. 1 (2013): 119–21.

Wharton, Amy. *Working in America: Continuity, Conflict, and Change*. 3rd ed. New York: McGraw-Hill, 2005.

White, Geoffry D., and Flannery C. Hauck, ed. *Campus, Inc.: Corporate Power in the Ivory Tower*. Amherst, NY: Prometheus Books, 2000.

White, Kathleen M., and Ann O'Sullivan. *The Essential Guide to Nursing Practice: Applying ANA's Scope and Standards to Practice and Education*. Silver Spring, MD: American Nurses Association, 2012.

Whitehead, Ann. "The Gendered Impacts of Liberalization Policies on African Agricultural Economies and Rural Livelihoods." In Razavi, *Gendered Impacts of Liberalization*, 37–62.

Whitehead, Phyllis B., Robert K. Herbertson, Ann B. Hamric, Elizabeth G. Epstein, and Joan M. Fisher. "Moral Distress Among Healthcare Professionals: Report of an Institution-Wide Survey." *Journal of Nursing Scholarship* 47, no. 2 (2014): 117–25.

Wilensky, Harold L. "The Professionalization of Everyone?" *American Journal of Sociology* 70, no. 2 (1964): 137–58.

Williams, Christine L., Chandra Muller, and Kristine Kilanski. "Gendered Organizations in the New Economy." *Gender & Society* 26, no. 4 (2012): 549–73.

Williams, Peter John. "Valid Knowledge: The Economy and the Academy." *Higher Education* 54, no. 4 (October 2007): 511–23.

Wilson, Lynda, and Marsha Fowler. "Leadership Needed to Address the Global Nursing and Midwifery Workforce Shortage." *Nursing Outlook* 60, no. 1 (2012): 51–53.

Winter, Gibson. *Elements for a Social Ethic: The Role of Social Science in Public Policy*. New York: Collier-Macmillan, 1966.

Wittig, Monique. "On the Social Contract." *Feminist Issues* 9, no. 1 (1 March 1989): 3–12.

Woods, Cynthia Q. "Evolution of the American Nurses Association's Position on Health Insurance For the Aged: 1933-1965." *Nursing Research* 45, no. 5 (1996): 304–10.

Wynia, Matthew K. "The Short History and Tenuous Future of Medical Professionalism: The Erosion of Medicine's Social Contract." *Perspectives in Biology and Medicine* 51, no. 4 (2008): 565–78.

Yarling, Roland R., and Beverly J. McElmurry. "The Moral Foundation of Nursing." *Advances in Nursing Science* 8, no. 2 (1986): 63–74.

Zakaria, Fareed. *In Defense of a Liberal Education*. New York: W.W. Norton & Company, 2015.

Index

H

I

J

K

L